MW01172547

The Commodity of Time

A heartfelt caregiver's
unexpected journey with her
mother through illness, cancer,
and everything in between.

a memoir by

LIZANN GRUPALO

Copyright © 2023 Lizann Grupalo

All rights reserved. No part of this publication may be reproduced or transmitted in any form or by any means, electronic or mechanical, including photocopy, recording, or any information storage and retrieval system, without permission in writing from the publisher.

Printed in the United States.

Cover and book design by Asya Blue Design.

ISBN Paperback: 979-8-9892789-0-9
ISBN Hardcover: 979-8-9892789-1-6
ISBN E-book: 979-8-9892789-2-3

AUTHOR'S NOTE

The events and experiences that follow are all true. I have not changed the names, identities, or other specifics of individuals to preserve the accuracy and integrity of the story. It also serves as a way to honor the doctors and nurses who played such an integral part in my mother's journey.

This story first started as an online blog in 2013, designed to serve as a gateway of communication with family and friends. I would write and publish daily posts while in the hospital. At home, the posts would occur a little less frequently, providing updates with Mom's story unfolding over the course of a year. This book includes the blog posts and other experiences which were originally omitted from the blog posts, respecting my mother's request at the time. There is truth in the telling and this story reflects the true essence, mood, and spirit of how this journey unfolds.

Dedication

To my mom, Dolly Grupalo, who has proven that together, we can weather the storms, fight the hard battles, celebrate the little wins, and do so with dignity, grace, and a little laughter along the way. Your courage, strength, and unwavering faith is an example from which we should all live by. Thank you for not giving up.

ILYMTT

To all caregivers who selflessly give of themselves to provide care, comfort, support, love, and understanding. Know that you are the angels on the ground making a difference in every life you care for.

"Time is a precious commodity and it must be used carefully and judiciously." –T.D. Jakes

"You have to accept whatever comes, and the only important thing is that you meet it with the best you have to give." –Eleanor Roosevelt

CONTENTS

INTRODUCTION

The intention in telling this human interest and personal story is to inspire and engage other caregivers and patients. As you navigate through the medical system and world of illness, may the words that follow provide insight and a lighted pathway on gathering accessible information, assessing options, and having a resolve in a quest for the answers that I worked so diligently to find. Working against the clock, my research was fast and furious. Time was certainly not on our side. Decisions had to be made swiftly about doctors and treatments. There was no time to sit back with a luxurious "wait and see" attitude.

In every situation, there are critical choices to be made. Often, however, the choices we face may not be desirable and the options even less so. I have always been a firm believer that inaction is also an action. If given the chance, my preference is to be action-oriented and in the driver's seat as often as possible. In order to take action in this battle against cancer, I needed to understand the cards my mother had been dealt. Being diagnosed with Stage 3 ovarian cancer required her to reevaluate her life and make some very difficult choices in a very short amount of time. The clock was ticking – loudly. One thing I knew for sure, my mother would need a "Special Ops" team in place to help her navigate through this time of her life – however long or short it would be. And I became determined to take the lead role in that responsibility and everything it entailed.

Perhaps this story will alleviate some anxiety, provide a few laughs, and help guide you to finding the right balance and plan of action for your road map through illness – including how to find the right doctor, determining the right course of treatment, understanding how diet will affect your recovery, and how one's spirituality can make a difference in healing. May it open your eyes, get you thinking in new ways, and provide you with the courage to ask the tough questions surrounding proper health care. Whether for yourself or a loved one, the journey may certainly be bumpy with unexpected blinding twists and turns along the way. But isn't that life?

The reality of death came knocking on my mother's door. Overwhelmingly, my inner voice called out to me, "Whatever you do, don't open that door!"

Through your own personal journey, whether it be a road map through cancer or navigating another illness, may you find the strength and resolve to find answers to your questions and fight the battle.

Through the tears, may you find laughter. Through the anger, may you find peace within. On such a path of the unknown, may you take control and live life on your terms, just as my mother has so gracefully done. And may you choose to see a light at the end of the tunnel and reap the benefits of a life well-lived surrounded by loving family and friends. Isn't that what this journey through life is all about?

PROLOGUE

In the upscale little enclave of Yountville, California is Pancha's, a dive bar of national notoriety. This non-descript, sand-colored wood shack is the ugliest building in town, but comes alive with a revolving door of customers. For the stories just ask Rose, the bartender and owner. She and her family have been here since the place was built in 1957. And nothing ever happens in this bar without Rose knowing about it.

One quiet fall evening of 2013, the Yountville Trolley transported a group of spirited ladies all dolled up in a colorful rainbow of feather boas to make their entrance into Pancha's. Nothing they did was ever less than grand or short on energy. And leading the pack was my mother Dolly, intent on celebrating her 75th birthday in style. With her entourage of 15 girlfriends in tow, they lit up this place.

Originally built as a beer bar and card room, the tobacco-stained walls were plastered with beer signs and thick smoke hovers over the pool table. The stench of stale beer permeated through the room. The bar stools were tattered to bits, resembling a sofa chair's exposed stuffing. The crowd was a mix of workers just grabbing a beer after a long day out in the sun-drenched vineyards, locals from the Veterans Home, and a few buttoned-up executive types looking to escape the office. A gentleman in the crowd offered up a round of drinks. As the feather-toting ladies circulated through the room with their drinks, Rose was tussling to help my mother climb up on the bar. With the jukebox playing, my mother, Dolly, broke out into a little soft shoe tap number and "shuffles off to Buffalo" to cheers from the crowd. Mom had reached a new low – or high, depending on how you look at it. In all these years, I had no idea she wanted to dance on that bar.

Instinctively, I knew something was wrong and would soon discover the inspiration for her rogue, out of the ordinary behavior. My suspicions were further confirmed when I saw a photo in print, making the social page of the *Yountville Sun* newspaper. There it was for all to see front and center – Mom dancing on the bar.

A late-stage ovarian cancer diagnosis propelled my mother to revisit her bucket list. It pushed me, however, into action of a different sort. My Type A personality kicked into overdrive. I appointed myself "General" of our little family's Special Ops team. My "to do" list was soon completed – quit my job, vacate my house in Las Vegas, return home to California, and move in with my parents. My new employment title was "Caregiver." A Scorpio to

the core, my fierce loyalty and ready-to-take-charge attitude rose to wage war against the disease. At the same
time, however, anxiety consumed me. I had absolutely no
idea what I was doing. There was no study manual on
navigating the world of cancer or how to be a caregiver.
Not one with a propensity for gambling, I laid it all on the
line here. This book is my story of how betting big became
a game changer and an unexpected return trip home.

CHAPTER 1

A LIFE-CHANGING DIAGNOSIS

I t was the first week of October 2013, and I was on a business trip in Albuquerque. As I was just about to walk into a meeting, I heard the ping of a text message come through on my iPhone. With a quick glance, I noticed that it was a text from Mom.

"Why would she be texting me?" I muttered with a faint sigh of frustration.

This was so out of character for her. She preferred to chat on the phone.

"It's just so much more personal," she would always say.

The text message was short and concise.

"Nan, the test results are in, and they are positive for ovarian cancer."

Feeling lightheaded and dazed with confusion, I immediately made a move to dial Mom's number…but then stopped. Isn't that why she just texted me? To create some space between us? She didn't want to discuss it – or couldn't – at least not at this moment.

With crushing sadness and a heavy heart, I looked up into the clear blue sky as the sun radiated an intensity and heat that helped dry my welling tears. All I could do was take a deep breath, try to regain my composure, and compartmentalize the devastating news as I proceeded to walk into the meeting.

Up to this point, Mom was the picture of health. Rarely sick, she never took medication and was living a very active and dynamic lifestyle. During the day she played on a tennis team and by night "Dolly's Dancers" were tap dancing to their hearts' content and getting their cardio in. All the ladies were "of a certain age," covering every decade from the 40s through the 80s. Over time, they grew a loyal following, earned a reputation for putting on a great show, and performed locally and throughout the San Francisco Bay Area. They were a hot ticket item in town and Mom's dance card was full! For having just turned 75, she hardly seemed her age. In fact, I often forgot that she was a "senior citizen" and could cash in on all the AARP discounts.

Although not a senior citizen yet, I was well aware of the shrinking gap and that I lagged not far behind. It wasn't that long ago, or so I liked to think, that I was in my 20s listening to and heeding my father's advice. One of his life lessons was encouraging my brother and me to never be afraid to leave home for the right career move. Taking those words to heart, that was precisely the path I followed. I left home, never looked back, and took advantage of every opportunity as I moved up through the ranks of the wine world. The adventure began in Sonoma, traveled south to Los Angeles, north to Monterey for an MBA, back to Southern California, and then over to Las Vegas. There was a detour to Toronto (for love and marriage), and then a one-way return ticket back to Las Vegas (because of a heartbreaking divorce).

With the passing time and accumulated life experiences, my intentions and focus had become laser-sharp and in tune with what I deemed as the most important priorities in my life. Fully invested in the commodity of time, I chose to cultivate meaningful relationships of a profound love and appreciation for my family, especially my mother. The sacrifices she made to provide for her family were certainly much better understood. With her strong work ethic, Mom always worked two jobs – as a nurse and as a mother. When we were young, it was working the night shift at the hospital on weekends so she could be with us kids during the week after school. Sundays were reserved for "time with Pop" and always began with Mass at St. Mary's College. So often I wondered if the church parishioners thought I was motherless due to her absence week after week. As a faithful Catholic and member of the St. Perpetua Church Guild, she found her time with God elsewhere. In my late teens, Mom worked a job I knew she disliked – as an occupational health nurse in a glass factory – to help pay the bills and make ends meet. College for two kids just 14 months apart in age was looming right around the corner. The fabric of Mom's DNA was exemplified over the years by her incessant work ethic and resilience to life's challenges. She was adept at making bad situations better and somehow always managed to find the silver lining.

BACK IN 1975, I REMEMBER one evening after a hard day's work for Mom and a long day of school for me. We were driving to my first ballet class. At dusk, the back roads were dark and tension in the balmy night air was high. At Mom's urging, we were venturing out to try something new. She focused on the positive, while I was focused on my nerves. My sullen, scowling 10-year-old self wanted no part of it. After a tense 30-minute drive in silence, we arrived only to quickly determine we were at the wrong location. This was a house – not a ballet studio. Apparently, the studio had moved just a few weeks earlier and we somehow missed the memo. Well before the invention of smartphones and the internet, we were on our own to figure it out. Somehow Mom persevered and found the ballet studio without any help from me. And now we were late. With anxiety at an all-time high, my meltdown moment had arrived.

"Mom, I don't want to go," I cried. "I don't want to take a ballet class. Please don't make me do this."

But she calmly ignored my tears and negative attitude

and proceeded to walk me into the class. Mom had nerves of steel and a resolve that was unmatched with her courage of conviction.

As the big, heavy wooden door creaked open, we stepped into another world. Inside was a charming dance studio, a softly lit room with little white lights twinkling around a big bay window. It was warm and inviting, but I hadn't quite figured that out yet. As we entered, the entire class turned to look at me. In my bright pink sleeveless leotard, pink tights, and pink ballet slippers, I gasped. A class full of elegant young dancers stared back at me from their smartly dressed uniforms – traditional black leotards with pink tights and pink slippers. I clearly stood out from everyone else when all I wanted was to blend in. Before my melt-down could escalate further, Susie Edgren, the teacher, approached me. With a sincere, heartwarming smile and comforting words, she encouraged me to join the class. As Pachelbel's Canon in D filled the room, my anger and anxiety quickly dissipated and at that moment I forgot I was different from everyone else. Mesmerized, the music and movement permeated through my bones and into my soul.

After class, on our drive home, I was beaming and couldn't stop giving Mom the play-by-play report of everything I had learned. I absolutely loved it, gave her a big hug, and thanked her for making me go.

Beyond all the tears and drama, Mom must have been smiling and whispering to herself, "I knew you'd love it."

By all accounts, I knew that looking into my mother's hazel eyes was the only way I would fully understand the state of her well-being, both physical and mental, since her diagnosis. I would see through the armor and assess her level of strength and fragility. Two weeks after receiving that text message, I would get my wish on October 17, 2013. An initial consult with a surgeon was scheduled and I would fly up to Northern California for the day. Since Mom's diagnosis, this would be our first family get-together – my parents, my brother, and me. I suspect that Mom was in some way relieved that we were meeting on neutral ground in a doctor's office. There would be a buffer – nurses and doctors circulating nearby to thwart any emotional outburst that may otherwise have occurred. Did I mention that we are an Italian family and emotions run deep?

I was the last to arrive at the Cypress Women's Cancer Treatment Center and greeted everyone with a soft and slightly reserved hug. It felt like I was just going through the motions. To Mom's credit she was stoic and kept it together, although I knew it wasn't easy for her.

She shot me a look of, "Don't you dare ruin my makeup and cause me to make a scene here."

As far as appearances go, I thought she looked the same. Or did she? Discreetly, I observed more acutely, dissecting her appearance from head to toe. She looked puffy and swollen. Her face was plump, she looked tired, and the twinkle in her eyes had disappeared. Her body language suggested resignation to accept whatever hand fate had dealt her. The fighting warrior spirit was nowhere to be found. As I tried to peer into her soul, I could tell she was temporarily shut off to all. For the time being, I would let it be. Self-preservation, I concluded. So, I chose to take a back seat and vowed to just be present…to listen and observe during the next few hours we would spend together.

ALONG WITH AN INCREDIBLY CARING and nurturing side, Mom was also the enforcer. We had rules to abide by and my brother and I always knew just how far we could push. There were always consequences to our actions, and we learned that lesson the hard way on numerous occasions. Often, we'd find ourselves in trouble after a long day of school when our pent-up energy needed to be unleashed. It didn't take long for law and order to prevail. The wooden spoon would always get our big, brown-eyed attention until one day my brother decided to match Mom's wits. Running through the kitchen and around the table, he somehow managed to grab a schoolbook, put it in his pants, and temporarily avert a backside spoon spanking. From then on, the spoon went into disciplinary retirement and would only reappear to stir the pasta sauce.

In conjunction with her influential guidance, Mom also had tremendous energy, was athletic, and proved to be our #1 fan. Afternoons were often spent exerting physical prowess, with us playing dodgeball, basketball, or roller-skating in the back yard. For fear of missing out, she attended all of our sports games and after school activities. We'd also venture out for bike rides or head over to the local high school courts for a game of tennis. And at the end of the day if we still had too much energy to burn, we were instructed to run around the house three times. This involved jumping hedges and trying to beat my brother to the finish line just as Mom was serving dinner. From childhood through adolescence and into adulthood, those meaningful shared bonding experiences are forever etched in my memory. A woman of great faith, Mom always stood her ground and never wavered in her beliefs even when she and I didn't see eye to eye. And through the countless peaks and valleys as life unfolded and I challenged her to the core, she never abandoned me. Whatever the challenge, she met it head-on with grace and diplomacy.

OVERNIGHT, I WAS MOONLIGHTING as a project manager to cancer. With the revelation that Mom now had a late-stage cancer diagnosis, it didn't take long for me to devise a game plan. Back from Albuquerque, the first weekend in October was spent in absolute solitude. Sitting at my desk on a quiet Saturday morning, with pen to paper I began to consider and list all the possible scenarios, noting the respective pros and cons. In essence, I treated it like another business problem that needed to be solved. Only this was different. It was life-threatening and personal. Certain actions would derive specific consequences and required further analysis and in-depth evaluation.

Initially, I seemed to have more questions than answers. How would my involvement affect each situation? Could I make a difference? Would I be a help or hindrance? What would this do to our mother-daughter relationship? Did Mom want to live and put up a fight? How did my parents collectively want to handle the situation?

One by one, ideas and options were flushed out in a chronological order and explored – research surgeons and hospitals, make appointments with doctors, seek second opinions, determine a course of action (surgery vs. no surgery), chemo vs. alternative treatments (whatever they may be), and where to have surgery or chemo (if that was the chosen path). One question led to another until pages were filled with notes. Drafting a timeline of my proposed action plan was a hard reality check. Could I be the life support for an indefinite amount of time whereby all normalcy would cease to exist in our lives? That was certainly a loaded question.

The day passed well into night. Exhausted from the mental workout, I collapsed into bed and slept solidly on it that night. Sunday morning was fully leaded with a caffeine-induced proper follow-up. Notes were reviewed, assessed, and a plan of action confirmed. In no short order, my "to do" list was written:

1. Quit job.

2. Move home (for as long as necessary).

3. Schedule and attend all meetings and doctors' appointments.

4. Encourage Mom to create and accept her action treatment plan.

5. Implement the plan.

6. Get Mom through surgery, treatment, and on a fast track to recovery.

Making the presentation and closing the deal would require my best performance. In my heart, I knew what to do. And in my mind, there was never a doubt. This proposed plan was covert and was never discussed with anyone other than my brother, Joe. Together we formed a unified front and a Special Ops team. For me to quickly depart Las Vegas and return home, I would need the support of my closest friends.

How long would I be gone? One month or six months?

Who would check on my house?

What about the mail?

How about my car?

The unknown variables were endless.

Expressing her deep concern, my closest friend, Carla,

confronted me about this life-altering upheaval.

"Are your parents asking you to come home?" Carla tactfully inquired.

"No," I gently responded. "That's not the case. My parents would never ask or expect that of me – to give up my life, interrupt my career, and come home to be a caregiver."

Always exhibiting a warm and heartfelt older sister mentality, Carla didn't disappoint as she reassuringly pointed out, "Lizann, I will be here for you. And I will do whatever I can to help you get home to be with your family."

Late Sunday afternoon, I nervously picked up the phone and called home. I knew my parents would be there – Pop watching the NFL football games on TV and Mom puttering around the house. Seeing my 702 number, Mom answered the phone promptly. It was a common occurrence for us to speak often, even daily. There was nothing unusual in this call except the hesitation in my voice. Sensing that this was different, Mom let me take the lead.

"So, how are you doing? Are you feeling ok?" I quickly asked, making small talk before diving deeper. "Can you fill me in on the updates from the doctors and the test results?"

In a matter-of-fact tone that you might expect from a doctor, Mom provided the synopsis with a steeliness and a hint of detachment. She spoke as though she didn't have the starring role in this nightmare.

Suspecting this was a defensive move to keep the floodgates from breaking open, I pushed onward...not giving her the chance to pull back.

"Mom, can you get Pop on the phone, too? I have a proposal that I want to discuss with both of you."

Eerily silent, the few seconds it took for my father to pick up the phone were incredibly uncomfortable. Hands trembling, I moved the phone to my other ear. Positioning myself upright in the chair to command my presence through the phone lines, it was time for the sales pitch. My mind was racing with anxiety. How were my parents going to react? Would they really listen to my plan, or would they dismiss it? What would I do if they rejected my idea? Ignoring those lingering thoughts, I fixated on moving this dialogue forward so that I could get into my flow.

"The reason I called tonight was to let you know that I have given the recent developments some serious thought. If you are in agreement, I would like to come home and help you both out. I know it's going to be a very long haul, but I'm prepared to go the distance. I would like to quit my job, come home, and be a caregiver to help you get through this."

Silence. And more silence.

"Helloooo? Are you guys still there?"

In a broken, wavering voice, Mom said, "Are you sure you want to do this? What about your job and your house?"

Sensing they were caught off guard, I could practically hear their minds spinning in the stillness as they tried to process my words and the weight they carried.

Immediately, I perked up and went in for the close.

"This is exactly what I want to do. And you both know I don't love this job. I've got it all sorted out. Carla, Chris, and Kristine said they will watch over my house and car while I'm away and take care of anything else in Las Vegas. Let me come home and help you get through this. As for work, I will revisit that when the time comes. I really am in the perfect position to help."

Once the shock subsided, my parents were extremely appreciative of the offer...and it didn't take long for the negotiations round to begin.

"Which room would you want to stay in? Nonni (my grandmother) is in the cottage, so you would have to stay in the house with us."

And so it went. As the minutes passed, the conversation continued to evolve and my parents were officially onboard with the master plan. The deal was done. Breathing a huge sigh of relief, I knew that in time, the next steps would gradually and naturally unfold. To manage this transition into unfamiliar territory, I would focus on being present and taking it one day at a time. As my Italian great uncle Netto used to say, "inch by inch." Worrying about the future had no place to occupy my thoughts now. It was all about survival and redirecting the energy to my mother.

Rarely do opportunities arise that allow us to step up and make a significant difference in someone else's life. In my case, maybe those opportunities had been there all along but were overshadowed by my inability to recognize them. With a clear vision, I could now give back to Mom in the way she had always given to me. Since the day I was prematurely born, when we were both fighting for my life, the strength and bond of our collective struggle for survival would be tested yet again. Now, during my mother's darkest hour, I would help guide her every step of the unknown way.

So here I am, late 40s, divorced, and about to move back home to live with my parents. This was never part of the well-thought-out game plan I had for my life. What the hell happened and how did I end up here?

CHAPTER 2

A REUNION WHILE
TROUBLE IS BREWING

Within weeks of receiving her diagnosis, Mom's zest for life would come to a screeching halt. Only later did I get the complete story.

Not feeling like her normal self for a few months, the most noticeable change was her tennis skirts getting tighter around the waistline. Mom figured at her age she was just overindulging in her beloved carbs (a good Midwestern girl at heart) and alcohol (preferably champagne) and needed to cut back. She felt full, would get short of breath, and found it uncomfortable to move around the tennis court. Those were the first warning signs. In the back of her mind, she contemplated that it was something more serious. Multiple visits to her primary care doctor at the time, did not provide any answers, only frustration to say the least.

After Mom explained her symptoms, the doctor pounded on Mom's abdomen trying to get "some action."

"There's nothing to be concerned about," she said. "Go home and take a laxative or some Milk of Magnesium and see if that helps."

It was a Friday afternoon and if nothing progressed, then a trip to the ER was recommended. The weekend came and went without any change. Bypassing a trip to the ER, a looming feeling still nagged at Mom.

Finally, after a few more weeks had passed without a diagnosis from her primary care doctor, Mom took matters into her own hands and made an appointment with her gastroenterologist. One of the many things I've always credited my mother with is having the sense to know when something isn't quite right. Perhaps it's in part due to her career as a Registered Nurse that had her well-trained in the world of health, medicine, and listening to your own body. In this instance, it served her well. She followed her instincts and went in for a second opinion with a doctor she trusted. On October 1, 2013, Mom met with Dr. Freeto. He expressed immediate concern and scheduled various tests and a CT scan for the following day.

With results in hand, Dr. Freeto delivered sobering words.

"We have trouble here and a major problem, Dolly," he explained to my parents as he scanned the results once more.

Although he never mentioned the word "cancer," she knew.

The hits kept coming as Mom learned she had Stage 3 ovarian cancer that had spread to all her major organs except her lungs. Dr. Freeto showed my parents the image – it looked like the night sky, only the stars were brightly shining cancerous tumors. The entire abdominal cavity was brimming with cancer.

"It's all throughout your body," he pointed out.

Time was now a precious commodity that could not be wasted, and they were swiftly ushered a few blocks over to make an appointment with Dr. Dugan, an oncologist.

As Dr. Dugan reviewed the charts and scans with my parents he murmured compassionately, "It's like you've been hit with an atomic bomb. And no one ever signs up for this."

Forty-eight hours later and adding a new doctor to her contact list, a blood test was ordered and Mom soon learned all about elevated CA-125 markers.

I don't recall my parents ever asking me to lie, except for now. They were drawing me into their web of deceit with my grandmother, one of the most beloved and special people in my life. My paternal grandmother, Nonni, as we called her (our iteration for "nonna" in Italian) lived in the cottage next door to my parents and ours was a very special and unique bond. My parents were now asking me to deny the truth to a woman whom I respected and loved. She ranked right up there with my mother.

"Nan, you can't let Nonni know why you are here visiting," my mother pleaded. "Just tell her that work brings you to town more often now. If she finds out what's going on, this will just kill her."

Following my mother's directive, I kept the secret with one lie covering for another.

Meanwhile, my dad, normally a prankster and one who likes to joke around and make light of a delicate situation, went quiet and reverted inward to what I assume were his own private thoughts. He would move quietly through the house as though he were a guest. Again, not normal behavior for my Italian father. Often, I would turn to easy conversation and common ground.

"Pop, what football games are on TV this weekend? Anything worth watching?"

He would rattle off the schedule to which I would reply, "Just don't ask me to watch the cheaters", as I've frequently referred to the Seattle Seahawks (in reference to Pete Carroll's illegal recruiting from his days at the University of Southern California) and the New England Patriots (in reference to Bill Billicheck's "spying scandal").

Those few words, like clockwork, would always get him riled and worked up, voice raised with Italian hands flying in the air as he defiantly explained his perspective.

It was our usual football banter. Except now, he wasn't fighting back. He just let it go and so did I. Watching sports on TV was and still is an integral part of our cherished father-daughter time. It just so happened that cancer hit our family during football season.

As conversations wavered toward Mom and her health,

Pop seemed caught off guard and preoccupied, as though he were enshrouded in a fog bank. I suspect he didn't fully understand the recent doctor to patient and nurse to patient conversations he was privy to or the ramifications of the hell they were both about to enter. Outside of his comfort zone, Pop was there for Mom when she asked him to accompany her to appointments. While I don't know the personal conversations that took place between them, my parents formed a unified front and chose not to reveal this diagnosis to anyone. With Mom's busy schedule still in full swing, there was another event on the horizon. In less than two weeks, Mom was scheduled to co-host her college nursing school reunion with her longtime friend and former classmate, Melba Rogoway.

THE STORY OF MOM'S DEPARTURE from her hometown of Rock Island, Illinois, cannot be told without mentioning Melba. You see, Mom, the third of four siblings, was the first to leave the nest. This did not go over well with my Midwestern Catholic guilt-infusing grandparents, especially my grandmother.

The memory is clearly etched in Mom's mind as, over many years, she has repeatedly recounted to me verbatim the one sentence that I suspect still haunts her today, "I hope you find whatever it is that you are looking for."

Ah, I know it so well as it, too, has been passed down

a generation to me. That passive-aggressive Catholic guilt creeps in and constantly serves to remind us of the unhappiness and disappointment we cause our parents. And somehow, we have to make amends in our own way to follow the dreams in our heart.

Back in those days, you just didn't abandon your parents and stray too far from home. Soon after graduating from nursing college, Mom and Melba made a pact and put their plan into action. I like to envision they were their generation's adventurous version of "Thelma and Louise." Their plan: get to Hawaii! The strategy: obtain contracted nursing jobs and work their way out West, saving money along the way. Landing in Palo Alto, California, they gained employment as nurses working at the Stanford VA Hospital.

Living in the same apartment complex in Palo Alto, my parents met one random afternoon in the laundry room. Ten cents short for the dryer, my father saved the day. And the rest is history. Taking a bit longer than anticipated (16 years to be exact), Mom did finally get her vacation in Hawaii. It just wasn't with Melba.

TIMING WAS CRITICAL NOW, as Mom and Melba were putting the finishing touches on their upcoming reunion. Ever since their 50th reunion, this group of 22 nurses and their spouses reconvened every two years. This year it would be in Yountville from October 14-16. While Mom was about to host her college classmates, my brother Joe and I were frantically working behind the scenes to get her an appointment to meet with a gynecologic oncologist surgeon. Making calls and sending emails to everyone in our expansive network of friends and colleagues, we were determined to get a meeting for Mom sooner rather than later. Joe worked his magic, pulled a few very big strings, and confirmed – at the very last minute – the date of October 17th to meet with a surgeon. The surgeon would make an exception to see us, and this was the only day available. We had to take it or leave it. So, we took it. The repercussions for Leah Rae Hyde, Mom's longtime friend and former roommate from nursing college who was visiting from Illinois, were hardest felt.

With the reunion in full swing, on Wednesday afternoon Mom approached Leah Rae.

Very direct and to the point, she stated, "Leah Rae, I'm sorry but you cannot stay with us tomorrow night. Something has come up."

Dumbfounded, Leah Rae was speechless. Suddenly, she found herself uninvited and stranded with nowhere to stay. The arrangement for Leah Rae to spend a few days with my parents after the reunion was rudely upended and there would be no further discussion. In the end, Leah Rae arranged for an early departure and flew home.

Overall, the reunion was a huge success, one joyous activity after another. No one suspected anything was seriously wrong. Weeks later Mom would finally break the news to Melba. Unable to manage the emotional strain of notifying friends and classmates, Mom asked Melba to share the update with all their friends and former classmates. Upon hearing Mom's diagnosis from Melba, Leah Rae immediately consulted her doctor and asked for an ovarian cancer screening test. The reluctant doctor finally gave in to Leah Rae's persistence and, to his surprise, her test results came back positive for an early stage of cancer. Who could have ever guessed that Mom's diagnosis would help one of her friends discover and avert her own cancer crisis?

Meanwhile, back at home and further complicating matters, my 97-year-old grandmother, Josie Grupalo's health was failing fast.

CHAPTER 3

A GRANDMOTHER'S LOVE

As the matriarch of our Italian family, Josie was a vibrant, strong-willed woman who lived a full life that always centered around the kitchen even when she lived with my parents. To her grandchildren, she was lovingly called "Nonni". Teeming with energy and never short on antics, she kept us all laughing and entertained. And I never met anyone who loved to play cards as much as Nonni. Her favorite game was 313 unless someone (that was always Mom) was up for a "road trip" to the nearest casino. The slot machines ruled over all else. And Nonni wasn't afraid to travel to expand her game – especially to Las Vegas where I conveniently happened to be living and working, focused on my career in the wine business.

With their great luck already brewing, I lived just a hop, a skip, and a jump away from the Red Rock Casino & Hotel. During all the years I lived and worked in Las

Vegas, I never gambled. It just wasn't my thing. However, I was more than happy to provide shuttle service and both Nonni and Mom latched on to take advantage of that opportunity. The schedule was that on my way to work, I would drop them off at the casino and at the end of the day I would pick them up.

Morning, noon, or night, those two were always ready for the slots. Nonni had her special brown leather money "pack" full of bills and ready for action. She wore it around her neck for safe keeping. There was no time to carry a purse! Usually, the planning conversation went something like this:

Me, "Ok, you guys are on your own this afternoon, but I'll be back at 9:00pm to pick you up. If you want to finish earlier, just give me a call on my cell phone and I will come and get you. Agreed?"

And they would agree. I knew my cell phone would never ring. As scheduled, I would show up at our pre-arranged time and (can you imagine?) they were never ready to leave.

Mom and Nonni, "Oh, is it already 9:00pm? We are on a roll and just got on these other machines! We're not quite ready to go yet. Why don't you grab a drink, sit down, and relax with us for a little while?"

Inevitably, time would pass...9:30pm, 10:00pm, 10:30pm...and there I would be after a long day at work, slumped over the machine, my head resting on the cool glass just waiting to hear them finally utter, "Ok, we are ready to go home now. We've got to pace ourselves and have energy for Round 2 tomorrow!"

These days, however, Nonni had very limited mobility and I sensed her growing frustration. Priding herself on being self-sufficient and active all these years, she now found herself reluctantly sedentary and dependent on others. Where was the joy in each day? Even reading was now a challenge for her. Judge Judy still provided daily entertainment, but even she was wearing thin. Day by day, Nonni's will to live slowly surrendered to her tired body.

A woman of faith, she would say, "I'm just waiting for my time to be called. I wish He would hurry up."

As winter approached, I could feel the weather turning dreary and cold. And I couldn't escape the internal dark cloud of sadness that hovered over the house and the cottage. Day in and day out, I honored my parents' request and never dared mention a word about Mom's cancer to Nonni. But it was a huge test of restraint for me layered with a tinge of betrayal. As witness to the extraordinary bond between my mother and my grandmother, I knew that Mom was considered more than just a daughter-in-law. In fact, Nonni often referred to Mom as "my angel." I know my grandmother had her suspicions, especially with my sudden, unusually frequent visits home. With a tilt of her head and eyes peering through me, she would just listen to my contrived explanations for coming home. I'll never know what she really thought because within just a few weeks on the evening of November 6, 2013, Nonni took her last breath.

As far back as I can remember, Nonni and I shared a unique bond that stood apart from everyone else. Our relationship was different, and everyone knew it was something special. Fondly, I remember standing in the kitchen, Nonni speaking her Piemontese dialect and me speaking the Tuscan Italian that I learned in high school and college. The fact that no one else in our family spoke or understood Italian granted us the freedom to have private conversations in the company of others.

"Ciao, Nonni." (Hugs and kisses here.)

"Come stai? Che cosa facciamo oggi? Possiamo fare una camminata?" *(How are you? What are we going to do today? Can we go for a walk?)*

I was also notorious for spinning into conversation not meant for my mom or my dad's ears (for example, expressing a negative comment on how I didn't want to eat the meat served at dinner that my mother had just spent hours preparing).

"Nonni, non mi piace questo carne. Non voglio mangiarla." *(Nonni, I don't like this meat. I don't want to eat it.)*

"Cara, se non vuole mangiare la carne, mangia la pasta." *(Dear, if you don't want to eat meat, eat pasta.)*

Suffice it to say, my smile was always bigger, my laugh heartier, and the sparkle in my eyes brighter when we were together. To Nonni's credit, she taught me about a woman's love of shoes (Ferragamo and Bruno Magli were her favorites) and how quality should always prevail over quantity. Stately at 5'8", she was impeccable in her dress, had a classic sense of style, was always appropriate, and knew her place.

As a child, some of my fondest memories were family weekends spent at my grandparents' Russian River summer home. It's where we gathered to escape the city heat. We were five grandkids in our motley crew – I was the eldest, followed by my brother Joe and our cousins Sara, Joe, and Colleen. Whether climbing the fig trees and running through the orchard, performing skits on the makeshift Redwood Forest stage, or picking berries for Nonni's blackberry cobbler, we were never bored. Mornings were best spent on the sun-drenched deck indulging in a big brunch that Nonni, Mom, and Aunt Toni had slaved over – eggs, potatoes, grilled onions, sourdough toast, and grilled skirt steak. And Nonno, my grandfather, always had the blender buzzing with the next batch of Gin Fizz. And brunch was always accompanied by the crooners on the record player – mostly Dean Martin, Frank Sinatra, and even Don Ho. Yes, Saturday mornings were made for "Tiny Bubbles."

One piece of advice that Nonni repeatedly doled out to us was, "Don't ever learn how to BBQ or make a drink. Leave that to the men to do."

And so she did. Oh, and her drink of choice? A Manhattan straight up, of course.

As I grew older, I discovered that while I did not like cooking, I sure did love being in the kitchen and cooking with Nonni. It was different with her. She made it fun, and everything was done with passion. Yearning for inspiration and her cooking secrets, I would barrage her with questions on her recipes for pesto, gnocchi, veal parmigiano, zucchini torta, antipasto, veal scallopine, polenta, and her infamous mushroom risotto. I quickly learned that she never measured ingredients (unless I begged her to, so I could write down the recipe). I wish I could say that I cook like that today, but I don't. It remains a distant memory of years gone by spending time with her in the kitchen, except for the recipe book she made for me called "Grandmother's Cooking Secrets."

It was always a fun adventure when we were going to Nonno and Nonni's house. Joe and I were always excited to get in the car and go. And upon our arrival, Nonni was always standing in front of the kitchen window looking out for us. Hearing Joe and I bound up the stairs, often two at a time, she'd greet us with big hugs at the front door. Immediately, we'd hit the bread drawer – second from the top. That's where we raided the Grissini breadsticks that would soon be wrapped with the sliced mortadella that was waiting for us. And every Thanksgiving and Christmas holiday was extra special, as I would get to help her make the homemade gnocchi. After the gnocchi, we would make the "bagnetto" – using the leftover ingredients from her homemade pesto. So simple and full of garlic. She knew it was my favorite and the reward for all the other hard work. My dad and I could eat bagnetto by the bowl, soaking it up with a fresh loaf of French bread!

But the greatest gift my grandmother gave me was opening my eyes to the expansive world that existed beyond the borders of my little hometown in California. She would speak endlessly of her travels and the world of possibilities. Nonni had a plan, and I would be the first participant.

At the age of 17, my high school graduation gift was a trip to Italy for just the two of us to visit the country and our family and relatives. As the first of the grandchildren to embark on this life-changing journey with her, I would set the course. I remember being so excited for my first adventure outside the United States, flying in a huge TWA airplane across the ocean to a foreign land where English was not the primary language. On a whirlwind group tour where everyone outranked me by 40+ years, we visited all the major sightseeing destinations. Here we wrote our own history together through Rome, Florence, Venice, Pisa, Milan, Naples, Sorrento, Capri, Verona, and Assisi.

Years later, Nonni and I would constantly reminisce and laugh about the afternoon in Rome when I kept the entire tour bus waiting because I'd lost track of time with a cute Italian boy I'd met at the hotel.

"Nonni, I'm just going for a ride around the block. I'll be back in time to meet the group for our departure."

"Ok, Lizann, but don't be late. We have to be on the bus at 3pm."

And off I went before she could utter another word. A hot summer afternoon in sundress and sandals, hair blowing in the wind, I jumped on the back of the moped and we sped away. Weaving in and out, navigating through the crowded, busy streets of Rome, Alfredo, a local Roman boy, wanted to show me his city. To this day, I've not enjoyed a better way to take in the sights of Rome!

As we pulled up to the hotel, I realized I was late. Very late. Everyone was on the tour bus glaring at me, including Nonni. As I quickly jumped off the moped to run up and get my tennis shoes, I turned back and shouted with a beaming smile.

"Grazie mille, Alfredo. Ci vediamo domani." *(Thanks so much, Alfredo. See you tomorrow.)*

Saving the best for last, our journey ended in Bonina, a small village in Piemonte, in the northwest part of Italy where Nonni's family is from. It was now just the two of us – time for a lesson in familial roots, understanding the heart and soul of our Italian family, and garnering a sense of the place from where we originated. It was finally time to meet aunts, uncles, cousins, and family friends.

New names expanded my vocabulary to family members – the matriarch Magnamina; aunts and uncles Elena and Rocco along with Eladae and Vladimir; and cousins Gabriella, Paola, and Fulvio. It was one big party day after day! There were festive gatherings morning, noon, and night. Some of my fondest memories include trying to communicate with Paola and Fulvio in my basic Italian, which often reverted to hand signals and my little pocket dictionary. My culinary skills were even tested with my cousin Gabriella when I attempted (at some ungodly hour of the morning) to bake what I called fancy bread – beautiful shapes of dough turned into delectable loaves of bread at her local bakery.

This was a life-changing trip where my world was forever changed. Nonni quietly inspired and encouraged my love of languages and a yearning for travel and discovery. The simple but bountiful lifestyle was now colorfully woven into the mosaic of what my future life could be.

Struggling to cope with my grandmother's death, my parents appeared almost despondent. It had become the perfect storm. I had no choice but to be strong and resilient for them. My time to mourn the loss of my grandmother would have to wait. While my heart ached, I didn't dare to stop and dwell on those feelings. More than ever, I needed to "cowboy up," as my Uncle Keith from Nebraska always says. It was time to pull myself up by the bootstraps, compartmentalize, and focus on how to keep Mom living.

CHAPTER 4

IN SEARCH OF A SURGEON

When your back is up against a wall and you are faced with the most challenging of times, that is when you dig deep and see what you are made of. How will you and those around you respond to a crisis? Who will be the one to step up to the plate and get involved? Who will make a difference? Who will lend a helping hand? Those are the questions I internally asked of myself and my family.

My brother Joe has always been consistently rock solid and level-headed. He is gifted with an ability to manage and reason with an incredible calm demeanor especially in the middle of a crisis. He was exactly the guy you want with you in the foxhole. He will have your back.

Through the years, he has proved this countless times. Never wavering, he has always been there for me when I needed it most. No surprise to report that he was a Captain with the El Cerrito Fire Department.

I have always said, "If I ever run into a problem, I want Joe to be the one to answer the call. I trust him with my life."

Once we both received the news of Mom's cancer diagnosis, we had a phone call that seemed more like a joint Chiefs of Staff strategy session. Methodically presenting a well-thought-out game plan, I sought his advice, guidance, and support. While we didn't always agree on everything, we both did have Mom's best interests at heart. Joe proved to be a great sounding board through each step of the journey and through some incredibly tense moments when I thought I was going to crack and fall apart, he was there to help me manage. Yes, he still had my back.

First thing Joe and I did was go online and start researching ovarian cancer. And naturally, Mom did the same. In hindsight, this probably wasn't the wisest thing to do. The amount of information on the internet was overwhelming and varied. My heart sank at reading the bleak survival rates and high rate of mortality. Right or wrong, good or bad, the information is all out there to sift through. The national statistics only invoked panic in all of us and I could feel my pulse quicken. Ovarian cancer was not in our vocabulary, and we all aimed to educate ourselves quickly. Mom was referred to Dr. Dugan, an oncologist, and the initial visit had her reeling from information overload. She barely had time to process all that was happening, much less think about making critical decisions regarding her life-threatening illness.

Dr. Dugan put it all in perspective as he expressed his concern, "Dolly, there is no time to waste. Your CA-125 marker is incredibly elevated at 2,388. A normal range would be below 35."

The numbers spoke for themselves. Could the situation be more dire?

As Mom would often hum from one of her beloved show-tunes, "Yes, we've got trouble, right here in River City." I have no idea what showtune that is from, by the way.

The silver lining was that I could see Mom had confidence in this doctor, and I knew that was incredibly important to her. Dr. Dugan then recommended that Mom meet with a surgeon as soon as possible. By the time she walked out of the doctor's office, she had a list of highly recommended doctors she never thought she would need – gynecologic oncologist surgeons in the Bay Area.

IT IS UNSETTLING THAT ALMOST every person I know is somehow affected and touched by cancer. Everywhere I turn, there is someone who has a story about a friend, loved one, or their own personal journey through cancer. Responding to this new role in our family crisis, I dove into researching, reading, and talking to anyone that could provide insight, offer advice, and help me navigate the world of cancer. The first line of defense put us in search of a surgeon.

Unbeknownst to me, I was working out in my local Las Vegas gym with a few people in the medical field. We never really talked about work other than a few words here and there. Literally, I had no idea of the amazing resources that were sweating, pushing their limits of strength and conditioning, and trying to catch their breath right next to me each week. Eventually, I discovered that one of my workout partners, Dr. Lynn Kowalski, is a well-regarded gynecologic oncologist. One of my other workout partners was Peggy Brennan, a trauma nurse. Another acquaintance outside of the gym, Sarah Ning, had worked for the Nevada Cancer Institute for many years. All three women were incredibly gracious with their time, answering all my questions and providing me with invaluable information. Enough cannot be said for utilizing one's resources. You just have to ask!

"Mom, now that you have this list of recommended surgeons," I explained on the phone from Las Vegas, "I've assigned us our first piece of homework."

Mom was eerily silent on the other end, but I knew that she was listening.

"Let's research these surgeons separately and pick the one that we each feel would be the best fit for you. Here is the list of questions I put together that we should reference during our research."

- "What traits do you want them to have?"
- "Do you care where they are located and how far away they will be?"

- "Do you want a more experienced doctor?"
- "Do you care where they attended medical school? Residency?"
- "What is their specialty?"
- "Have they won any awards?"
- "What are their hobbies?"
- "What do other patients say about them?"

Mom agreed to my plan and now had her first research assignment.

To keep us focused and on track, I suggested, "Let's regroup on a call at the end of the week to discuss our findings, thoughts, and selection."

Fortunately, living in the Bay Area of California allowed us to choose from highly skilled and renowned hospitals, medical facilities, doctors, and nurses. We reviewed the names of the recommended surgeons from UCSF Medical Center in San Francisco and John Muir Medical Center in Walnut Creek.

What a small world it was when I found out that Dr. Lynn Kowalski from my gym in Las Vegas actually knew one of the surgeons on the list. She had done her residency with Dr. Babak Edraki, a renowned and highly regarded surgeon in this field. Unbeknownst to me at the time, she had made a personal call to Dr. Edraki, providing a reference and alerting him that Mom may be reaching out for a consultation.

Conversations with Mom gradually became more candid as she offered up more opinions. She started to take ownership and dictate what she would and would not accept.

"Mom, as we start looking at surgeons, you also need to think about and identify the areas that you are most concerned about with regards to surgery, post-surgery recovery time, and follow-up treatment. We'll take it step by step and I'll follow your lead. But ultimately, the decisions will be yours to make."

We quickly discovered that many of the best regarded and renowned hospitals and cancer treatment centers required a plane and a pilot. These were what I called "GU" – geographically undesirable. And being "GU" was something I found to be of great importance to Mom. I hadn't really thought about distance and driving, but it repeatedly came up in our conversations.

"Nan, I want to be close to home. I don't want to fly anywhere, and I don't want to drive very far. What if something happens and I can't get to my doctors?"

Already feeling miserable and anxiety-ridden, she couldn't fathom having to manage a scenario filled with planes, trains, and automobiles. Opting to wage battle with cancer on her home turf, she chose a safe, comfortable, and familiar environment. Any decisions would need to fit within this parameter. I guess you could say she was hoping for a home field advantage.

Delving into my research on the surgeons, I tried to compile a picture of who they were and how they would fit with Mom. Could I find someone that she could not only trust and believe in to get the job done, but also bond with? Did I mention that Mom's always had very high standards? As a former RN, she knew what she was dealing with and needed to find a doctor who could communicate on her level. The surgeon who would win Mom's approval would need to be accomplished and confident; she needed someone who could not only deliver the facts, but who also had some bedside manners. Did I mention that Mom was also a stickler on manners?

At the end of the week, Mom and I got on the phone to discuss our findings. We had each narrowed down the playing field and made a final selection. Now I was curious to hear how well-aligned we were in our surgeon selection, and I was secretly nervous and hoping that we hadn't picked different surgeons.

"Mom, did you find a surgeon that you think will work for you?"

"Yes", she stated. "I found my surgeon – Dr. Dimitry Lerner. I reviewed his bio, looked at his schooling, read the patient reports, and even watched his interview on YouTube. He's young, but I think he's dynamic and has the drive and knowledge of cutting-edge technology."

Smiling to myself, I breathed a huge sigh of relief. Yes! We had picked the same surgeon. From what I could tell on paper, Dr. Lerner appeared to be the protégé to Dr. Edraki and the perfect surgeon for Mom.

His bio was nothing short of impressive, but what resonated with me was reading this line, "When not working, Dr. Lerner is training for the next Triathlon in the foothills of Mt. Diablo."

If he had the endurance and mental toughness for tri-athlons, then I figured he might have the right mental acuity to handle Mom and her impending complicated and difficult surgery.

The true test would come at a face-to-face meeting. One thing I do know from my short-term online dating experience, what you see on paper is not necessarily what you get in person!

What is he like in person?

What is his disposition?

More importantly, how does he interact with Mom?

These were all the little things I would be looking for in the initial consultation. With "the chosen one," I proceeded to learn more about the Cypress Women's Cancer Treatment Center where Dr. Lerner and Dr. Edraki were partners. Putting my sales skills to work, I went so far as to study up on each of the employees, learn their names and areas of responsibility...so that the minute I walked in the door, I would be able to identify everyone. The ultimate goal was to be on a first name basis with the staff, hoping that it might make a little difference in the level of care Mom would receive.

Navigating through doctors' offices and trying to book an appointment was certainly not without its challenges. For us, it was even more frustrating as we were racing against the clock. An initial call revealed a wait time of over a month for a consultation. In desperation, we knew we didn't have a month to wait. Joe, being ever so resourceful, made a few phone calls and, ultimately, called in a big favor from a friend. Somehow, he worked his magic. Before we knew it, Mom had an initial consult set for October 17, 2013. The moral of the story here is we didn't accept "no" as an answer and kept pushing forward to create a different outcome.

As a family, we all agreed to be present at the consultation and show strength in numbers and support for Mom. At the same time, I also wanted to ensure that we all heard the same message from the doctor. As Mom's Special Ops team, we all needed to be working from the same road map and moving cohesively in the same direction. Doing what was necessary, I adjusted my work schedule and hopped on a Southwest flight to Oakland for the day.

CHAPTER 5

A MEETING OF THE MINDS

Sitting in the quiet waiting room after greeting my family, I finally looked around. It was eerily silent, as we were the only ones in the waiting room. We had an appointment before normal office hours. A sparse room, there were more chairs than I thought there would be. Are there that many cancer patients requiring a gynecologic oncologist?

Amidst a forest of plants trying to invoke life that overflows here with cancer patients, I wondered how this day would unfold. My palms were sweaty (not a norm for me, by the way) as we waited to be called in to meet the doctor. At the appointed time, Mom was first led into a room for an initial private conversation with Dr. Lerner. Meanwhile, my dad, Joe and I were led into a small conference room. I noticed the room was bare, with just a few chairs and only a box of Kleenex front and center on the table.

Finally, Dr. Lerner and Mom entered the room and he

was just as I imagined – very young and handsome (an extra added benefit for Mom), soft-spoken, and gentle yet direct. He seemed to tread lightly as he assessed the room and the family he'd been dealt. There we were -- the Grupalo clan seated around a circular table, my parents in the middle flanked by Joe and me. With a file of Mom's lab reports and X-rays in front of him, he concisely delivered the results, diagnosis, and recommended course of treatment.

"The findings show you have fluid in the belly, spots on the abdomen, and an elevated tumor marker," he stated matter of factly. "We won't know how extensively the cancer has spread until we get into surgery."

The dialogue that ensued included words that didn't exist in my vocabulary. As I frantically took notes, my head was spinning.

Dr. Lerner continued, "The recommended surgical process would consist of extensive debulking surgery to remove all the tumors."

What does that even mean? I wanted to ask that question, but I refrained. And what an ugly word, by the way.

"There would be a laparoscopy hysterectomy (removal of the uterus, ovaries, and fallopian tubes), and possible surgery to remove a portion of the colon, lining of the abdomen (omentum), lining of the diaphragm, and spleen," Dr. Lerner added.

Was there anything left that wouldn't be removed? Where was the silver lining in all of this? Mom had always told me to look for the silver lining. In this case, I think it was debulked!

"Your time in the hospital is expected to be between 7-10 days."

The exact number would be 13 days.

"There will most likely be post-surgery in ICU for 1-2 days to accommodate the fluid shift. And approximately 6 weeks post-surgery, you will need to start chemotherapy. That course would run once a week for 18 weeks."

Once completed, the doctors would then do a follow up scan to reevaluate the results.

We continued to sit in silence and listen to the verdict, nodding our heads in understanding...or at least acknowledgement.

Dr. Lerner further stated, "We have a 70% success rate, but most patients will have a recurrence at some point."

"What's most important to note is the interval time between treatment and a recurrence. The more time that passes between treatment and a recurrence, the better."

Through all the tests and meetings with doctors, Mom learned her cancer was Stage 3. It was aggressive, fast spreading, and had already spread to other organs.

Mom admitted to Dr. Lerner and all of us that she was not keen on having surgery. She was adamant about finding out how far her cancer had spread to determine if surgery would even be worthwhile. Was it so far spread that they couldn't remove the tumors? Well, I thought, now's the time for the doc to step up and prove his worth to Mom.

I could see the wheels turning in her mind, "Here's your

first test and let's see what you have to say."

All of us turned from Mom back to Dr. Lerner.

And here is where I think Dr. Lerner earned one of his first stripes with Mom right away.

"We can do a PET scan and perhaps that will ease your mind and help to determine whether you elect to have the surgery."

I could see Mom relax just a bit. I liked him already and I knew that she did, too.

"However," he explained with clarity, "if you do not have this surgery right away, you probably won't live beyond a few months."

And there it was. That was the choice clearly spelled out. Silence hovered between us until he pushed forward.

"If you do opt for the surgery, you will need to do follow up blood work and an EKG one week prior to surgery. And we are looking at early to mid-November when there is an opening. Your surgery will be extensive and require a full day with both Dr. Edraki and me."

For Dr. Lerner, full-day surgeries were his Tuesdays.

Mom then went into what I call "nurse mode" and started her questioning, covering all the particulars and red flags that were front of mind for her. Clearly, she had given this thought and was prepared.

Interestingly, there were two points she was adamant about. Under no circumstances did she want a colostomy. I hadn't even thought that far ahead. But as a nurse, she knew what that would entail. I, on the other hand, had no idea.

The second point she drilled home was not to be on a ventilator. And what about the suctioning? (We later learned that you can request a scheduled sedation – NOT PRN.)

At the very least she made it known to Dr. Lerner what her trigger points were. We wouldn't know the outcome of these two stipulations until after surgery.

Family support was unequivocally front and center and for three of us – everyone but Mom – we voted in favor of having the surgery. But I certainly understood where Mom was coming from. Why go through hell if it can only extend your life a few months or so?

One point Mom clearly reiterated was her choice for quality of life over quantity. Who could blame her? I would have said the same thing.

But when you are the daughter, husband, or son, the only words you want to hear are, "Yes, let's put up a fight."

I wanted Mom to fight for her life like I was willing to fight for her. At this point, she was so overwhelmed and exhausted. I don't think she could wrap her mind around the idea of going through this ordeal. And she just didn't have the physical or mental energy right now. It was easier to just say no. But for Mom, there would be no easy cop out with her Special Ops team. We were in place and ready to help guide her through the darkness.

With all the cards now out on the table, I quickly realized that Mom was having a very hard time speaking. It finally hit home that her options were few and she didn't like any of them. Not exhibiting her normal take-charge behavior, I decided to step up and use this time to ask a few questions of my own. It was important for me to insert myself in the dialogue with Dr. Lerner and convey to him that I would have a central role in my mother's care.

Calmly and slowly, I placed my hands atop the binder on the table. This was filled with her lab reports, test results, doctors' lists, research notes, and two pages of my questions. Politely, I mentioned that I had a few questions I would like to ask. With his approval, I pulled my list of questions from the binder and proceeded down the list one at a time.

Prior to this meeting, I was fortunate to have spoken with my Las Vegas gym friends Lynn and Peggy who assisted me in putting together a list of appropriate questions. They included:

- What are your findings from the scan and test results?
- Is this curable through surgery and chemo?
- What is your recommended course of action for treatment?
- Who assists you in surgery?
- Do you send the tumor for molecular profiling?
- What are the benefits?
- Can you walk us through the process for the surgery?
- What is the estimated length of time in surgery?
- What is the estimated recovery time in the hospital?
- What is the estimated recovery time at home?

- How soon would you start chemo after surgery?
- Do you administer chemo (this is the only cancer field where surgeons can administer chemo)?
- Following surgery, what is the recommended chemo treatment?
- What do you recommend for diet post surgery?
- What are your thoughts on neo-adjuvant chemo?
- Is my mom a candidate for intra-peritoneal chemo?
- Can you do a BRCA test?
- What is your case load and how often are you in surgery?
- What does my mom need to do to be prepared for a successful operation?

I was relentless with my questioning and my family just looked at me wondering, "Who are you and what are you doing?"

About halfway through my barrage of questions, Mom reached out directly across the table and rested her hand on top of Dr. Lerner's.

She gave him a pat and said, "It's ok, she's just being thorough."

It was just the bit of an ice breaker we all needed as a hint of laughter filled the room. It may have seemed like the inquisition, but I was there to do a job. After Dr. Lerner respectfully answered all my questions, he reiterated his recommended course of treatment and suggested that Mom secure a surgery date before leaving the office today.

He further encouraged her, "If you decide you do not want to have the surgery after seeing the results of your PET scan, you can always cancel it."

As our meeting was wrapping up, I asked Dr. Lerner if we could have a word alone.

Stunned, everyone looked at me with a "Now, what are you doing?" stare.

Of course, I just dismissed them.

With my binder held closely to my chest, Dr. Lerner led me into an empty exam round down the hall. Standing about a foot apart, I looked him directly in the eye and began to talk about the woman he was about to add to his patient list (or so I hoped).

"I want you to know that my mother is so much more than what you see written on paper. She has a vibrant energy, engaging demeanor, and a love of life that's unmatched. She's athletic and very active – tennis player, tap dancer, party planner, and so much more! Her life is filled with a beautiful and close-knit family and friends. And there is a very special place in her heart reserved for her two grandchildren Gabriella and Dominic."

"Although she didn't exhibit these traits in your office today, she is an incredibly strong, determined woman and one full of faith. She is a tough mental competitor. She won't be an ordinary or average patient for you. She'll test you and require the best from you. But she is worth it. She is extra special and in time, you too, will come to realize this."

I will never know what impact, if any, that conversation had with Dr. Lerner. Taking advantage of the opportunity for a candid one-on-one conversation, I left no stone unturned and nothing to chance. It was all out on the table, and he listened ever so graciously. I remember my final comment was direct and to the point.

"My mother has done her due diligence and research. Among all the surgeons on the list, she chose you. And I agree with her choice. She has total faith in your ability, as do I."

"I promise you this – if you do your job, I will make sure we do ours. We will provide her with the best support network and be by her side every step of the way."

In closing, I sincerely thanked Dr. Lerner for his time and firmly shook his hand. We proceeded back to the room and rejoined my family where the meeting was quickly adjourned.

Upon saying our goodbyes, Dr. Lerner introduced us to Mojdeh Palmer, the office manager who was a gem and helped Mom set up a "tentative" surgery date.

As we walked out of the office, no one dared ask me about my conversation with Dr. Lerner. Completely drained and exhausted, we were mentally spent. Silently, I knew this was just the beginning of a path down Hell's Lane. So many questions were racing through my mind. Would Mom elect to have the surgery? Could she handle it? How would we manage? One thing was for sure – with time our true colors would be blazing bright – the good, the bad, and the ugly.

CHAPTER 6

A MATRIARCH'S PASSING

On October 23, the first order of business was the PET scan. There was a specific "to do" list and I was to make sure Mom was prepared – fast for six hours, don't eat or drink anything except water, drink 24 ounces of water within three hours of arrival, and wear comfy clothes with no metal. This scan would show Mom how far her cancer had spread and would be the driving force on whether she would elect to have the surgery.

The PET scan results were delivered:

Negative for any additional cancer found in her other vital organs.

While I don't know the thought process that Mom took in evaluating the pros and cons to surgery, one thing was clear. She knew she had 100% support from her family. We had her back on this. Collectively, we wanted her to fight and not give up. Clear as day, I remember the conversation at the round table with Dr. Lerner.

"Mom, we all want you to fight for your life," I said. "And we are all willing to change our lives and do whatever is needed to help you. Won't you please try? At least once? And if you decide later that you don't want to go through it again, we understand."

Little did I know what I was asking. Only much later did I discover that the debulking procedure is one of the most complex and difficult surgeries of all.

I don't remember the exact moment when Mom told me she would have the surgery, but that's probably because I couldn't think of the outcome any other way. A flurry of planning quickly ensued. Now that she had addressed the physical aspects of her cancer, my next step was to get her mentally prepared.

As I sought advice in dealing with Mom's cancer diagnosis, it was most often professional advice that I looked for – but at other times it was personal advice, derived from someone else's experience with cancer. The conversations could be technical – discussing the genetic makeup of cancer cells, how they spread, what surgery can do, what chemotherapy drugs were the best, and what the recovery process entailed. At other times, the conversations focused more on an "East meets West" philosophy – how to integrate the Eastern medicine viewpoint of collectively treating mind, body, and spirit with the best Western medicine. My inquiring mind wanted to also understand the benefits of mental preparation better. Could it make a difference and impact the healing process, emotionally as well as physically?

In my research, one of the books that I gravitated towards was Anti-Cancer: A New Way of Life by Dr. David Schreiber. It resonated with me on many levels, and I wanted to share this information with Mom. With her more traditional views on treating illness and disease, I tried to keep her mind open to the possibilities of adding a mental component to her fight.

"Mom, I really think you should read this," I pleaded.

The reality was that she was not going to read a book and especially one on cancer. Soon, I found myself providing her with a one or two-page document of "key points" from any publication that I found interesting. It was another way to keep her engaged in the process. In the meantime, while she was reading up on her mental preparation, I was back in Las Vegas giving my two weeks notice at work. Surgery was scheduled for November 13, 2013.

On October 29, I sent an email to all my friends and colleagues notifying them of my sudden move back to California. Was it temporary or permanent, they asked. I didn't know yet. All I could do was book a one-way ticket, pack a small suitcase, and hand over my house and car keys to Carla and Chris for safe keeping. My dearest friends were there for me in my time of need.

Besides offering their support and love, Carla and Chris promised to collect my mail, regularly check on the house, and keep my car running while I was gone. I literally left everything, walked out the front door, and locked it behind me. It would be another five months before I returned home to Las Vegas.

Around the same time, Mom slowly notified loved ones of her illness. She knew all the phone calls would be exhausting, so she opted to create and send "group" emails. She could then reach out to friends and family via phone on her own terms when she was ready to have those hard conversations.

Concerned about the communications overwhelming her, we started to brainstorm various ways to limit the exposure to what she could handle. Through Darlene Bevin, one of Mom's tap dancers, we heard about a website – www.CaringBridge.org. This would become the perfect solution to keep in touch with people near and far without having to expend energy on multiple phone calls or emails with the same update. What an amazing resource this is! And it saved us both, but for different reasons. I learned how to blog, provide updates, and even post photos. For Mom, it would soon become the one thing she looked forward to reading nightly in the hospital and beyond.

Initially, I began reading my commentary to her out loud each evening. Then it gradually progressed to include reading all the comments and loving wishes that friends were posting. It became an integral and positive focal point for Mom. It was a gentle reminder of all the friends, family, love, and prayers that were being sent to her. She was still connected to the outside world.

As we prepared for the upcoming surgery, I recruited

my 16-year-old niece Gabriella (aka Gab) and my 12-year-old nephew Dominic (aka Dom) to help Ammy (as they called Mom) make a "vision board" for her. This would become her visual lifeline – what she could focus on to get through the dark days in the hospital and beyond. I wanted her to see all the good that awaited her at the end of Hell's Lane. The goal was for Mom to believe that she could do and be all that was on her board. To personalize the board, I asked her a few questions.

"Mom, I've recruited Gab and Dom on a project. They are going to make a vision board for you."

She may have rolled her eyes at me at the time, but I ignored it. It was important to me to engage the grandkids, as I knew how important they were in Mom's life. Did I mention that Mom went so far as to pass on the opportunity to have an earlier surgery date due to a cancellation? She absolutely would not miss Gab's Senior Powder Puff Football Game at Carondelet High School. A good thing, too, as we got to witness Gab scoring the winning touchdown! I knew Mom would pay attention to anything that Gab and Dom created for her and that it would have profound meaning.

"Can you tell us what is most important to you right now?" I asked.

"What types of activities do you want to do when you feel better?"

"How do you want to spend your time?"

"What has the most meaning to you?"

"Is there anywhere you would like to go and visit?"

The answers were transformed through photos, words, and pictures as Gab and Dom created Ammy's vision board. We had decided to present it to Mom in her hospital room after surgery and we hoped it would accompany her home.

With Nonni's sudden passing, I flew home to California on November 11. Her funeral was scheduled for the following day, November 12, and the day before Mom's surgery. Barely unpacked, around 9:30pm that evening, when things were finally quieting down, Mom and I finally caught up.

Sitting on the edge of the bed, I asked, "Ok, Mom, I just want to make sure you completed the pre-op checklist from Dr. Lerner."

In a daze, she looked at me and I knew we were in trouble. Immediately, I went and grabbed her binder and flipped through it to find the requisition notes for the EKG and bloodwork that was to be completed one week prior to surgery. The week had come and gone and in taking care of Nonni, Mom had forgotten all about herself. Acting quickly, I called the doctor's office and asked the answering service to page Dr. Lerner and have him call me at home. Here we were already causing issues and Mom hadn't even entered the hospital yet. Well, I did warn the doc that nothing would be normal with Mom. Within 15 minutes, I received a phone call from Dr. Lerner.

In a hurried voice, I blurted out, "Dr. Lerner, I'm so sorry to call you this late at night. But I just arrived home in California and am with my mom reviewing her pre-op documents. She forgot to do her bloodwork and EKG tests. My grandmother just passed away, her funeral is tomorrow, and my mom has been preoccupied."

Finally, stopping to catch my breath, he could now get a word in. Calmly and patiently, he listened and then instructed me to have Mom go and get her the blood test done the next day after the funeral. He would take care of arranging the EKG for the morning of her surgery.

On Tuesday, November 12, we all gathered for Nonni's funeral at St. Joan of Arc Church in Yountville. An especially drab, overcast, and drizzly fall day compounded the emotional difficulty as my parents had to greet friends and loved ones who came to pay their respects. Incredibly poised as they greeted everyone, my parents displayed true grace and fortitude, as this was the first time seeing everyone since Mom's cancer diagnosis. Since the last time I had seen Mom, she had become increasingly more tired and uncomfortable. Perhaps it was a blessing that Mom had to leave right after the funeral service, which afforded her a little peace and quiet time alone. It was early evening before we got home and had to start thinking of tomorrow. We all retreated to our rooms and tried to get some sleep, as we had to be on the road early the next morning.

CHAPTER 7

A DAY OF RECKONING

In the pitch black of the early morning, we loaded our bags into the car and drove to John Muir Hospital in Walnut Creek. The only sound was the hum of the engine. Reporting in at 7:30am, it was an hour-long drive and one that my dad would get used to driving alone daily.

At this early hour, the hospital was hushed. To combat nerves, I opted for silence as Mom got checked in. She never was one for idle chit chat. Patiently and quietly, we sat in a small, non-descript waiting room. The nurse, one of many I'd see that day, called for Mom. It was time to go. As my parents shared a tender moment together, I walked ahead with the nurse. Mom had chosen me to be her pre-op guest and I would remain with her until she entered the Gates of Hell through the operating room.

As the nurses circled and made their rounds for blood work, charting, and all the other pre-op activities, they immediately took to Mom once they saw "Former RN" listed on her chart. They took her under their wing as one of their own and did everything to ensure her comfort. Mom even reminisced with them about the days she used to work in this hospital. Although it was years ago, she spoke fondly of the old wing. It was reassuring for me to know that this building still bestowed a level of familiarity and comfort for her.

As the ominous time drew near, Dr. Lerner appeared in his scrubs to check in and say hello.

"Dolly, I'm here to review and walk you through the surgical procedures that we will be performing today and there is some paperwork that we will need you to sign."

As Dr. Lerner spoke, I saw Mom start to get visibly shaken and upset. Lying on the gurney, her eyes darting back and forth, she was soon rubbing her hands incessantly. She was clearly agitated. While I understood he had rules and protocol to follow, I knew that the words only registered the impending visit to Hell she was about to be escorted into.

At some point in the dialogue, Dr. Lerner mentioned the word "colostomy" and "possible bowel re-sectioning" and that was the almighty trigger. The flood gates were now unleashed.

Mom immediately bolted herself upright and yelled at Dr. Lerner, "You absolutely promised me that I wouldn't need a colostomy. No! No! I told you that I wouldn't do this surgery if I had to have a colostomy."

Wet, hot tears streaming down her face, she continued to cry out, "You promised! You promised!"

Never had I seen my mother so vulnerable and emotional. Deeply unsettling, it touched me to the core and I nearly unraveled. My entire body now ached, and my heart broke into a million pieces as I internally contemplated, "Did I ask too much of her in having this surgery?"

Right now, I just wanted to hug her, comfort her, and make all the bad disappear. She didn't deserve any of this. Our reality was unforgiving and unchanging. And there was nothing I could do to alter the circumstances.

Trying to maintain my own state of calm, I softly whispered, "Mom, Dr. Lerner isn't saying that he has to do a colostomy. He just has to do his due diligence and go over all the possibilities."

With her nerves beyond frayed, she wasn't hearing me at all. Meanwhile, a pre-op nurse hurried over to administer Mom some sort of "let's-keep-her-off-the-ledge" medication through her IV.

From my chair, I looked up at Dr. Lerner who had somehow miraculously managed to maintain his composure during Mom's verbal lashing.

Pleading with my dark brown eyes, I gently uttered, "Dr. Lerner, you know how my mom feels about this. Please, just do everything you can so that she doesn't have to have a colostomy. I know you'll do your best. Thank you."

As he turned to go, I glanced over at Mom and thought to myself, "This really is not going well. Your doctor is about to go in with a toolkit of sharp knives to operate on you for nine hours and you just ripped him a new one."

But then again, I had warned him about Mom.

PRIOR TO MY DEPARTURE FROM LAS VEGAS, I received an incredibly thoughtful gift from my dear friend Chris Flatt. She had arranged for me to have a "reading" with a friend of hers, Christine, who is a psychic. Never advertising to the public, Christine operated discreetly and only by referral. She not only had an ability to cross over and communicate with our loved ones on the other side, but she could also see into the future.

"Lizann, your mom is going to be in the hospital and her surgery will go well. But she is going to have some sort of episode. I'm just telling you, so that when it happens you don't worry."

RATTLED, I SLOWLY MADE MY WAY DOWN to the waiting room to join the rest of my family – my dad, Aunt Beth (my mom's youngest sister), and her husband Keith. Joe would come later in the day. Not letting on to the fiasco that just transpired upstairs, I kept it light and told them lies.

"Mom is in good spirits and ready to fight," I declared.

Before ushering her into the OR, I gave Mom a little pep talk.

"Mom, you always tell me that your happy place is being at a babbling brook with your feet dangling in the water. Well, that's where you need to go right now. See the future you envision for yourself surrounded by your loving family and friends. You've got Gab's basketball and Dom's baseball games waiting for you. Fight for that. And I'll be here waiting for you. I love you."

She may not have heard a word I said, but for my own self-preservation I had to believe the positive messaging would somehow seep into her soul.

TODAY WAS THE OFFICIAL DAY MY CARINGBRIDGE blog was born. To preserve the integrity of this story, I've maintained the blog and, I've included supporting stories and commentary that I had initially, and often intentionally, left out. Before her surgery, Mom and I discussed the blog and what it should entail. Mom was adamant that I use restraint and not make this a "tell all story." I was not to mention the less than desirable aspects that she would encounter. I respected her wishes at the time, as I figured it was her way of trying to exert some control over the situation. She may not like it, but now I'm filling in the blanks to tell the whole story.

Wednesday, November 13, 2013
The Hospital

Here's to the beginning of this blog! I will do my best to keep you all updated as to the status of Dolly.

Thank you to everyone who was there for my grandmother Josie's funeral yesterday. I hope you know how much it meant to my mom during this difficult and challenging time to see all of you. Your kind words, love, and prayers for my mom are so very much appreciated!

Mom went into surgery this morning around 9:30 am at John Muir Hospital. Dr. Lerner had finished another surgery early, which made me happy to hear that he was warmed up, ready to go, and on his "A" game for my mom! One thing I know is that she is in GREAT hands! This is a state-of-the-art hospital with amazing surgeons and nurses all around! Side note: did you know they even have valet parking here? And an afternoon pianist to keep us company while we wait to get a surgery update? Very impressive!

NO VISITORS WILL BE ALLOWED AT THE HOSPITAL DURING HER STAY. This is my mom's wish, and we would greatly appreciate it if you respect her wishes until further notice. You all have my phone number in case you need to reach me. Otherwise, I'll continue to provide frequent updates.

Have you ever been in a hospital waiting room for 11 straight hours? I was climbing the walls with nowhere to roam except the cafeteria. My stomach was in knots all day and my butt was sore from sitting so long. The silver lining here is that this is a beautiful hospital. Split into two large rooms, there are high-vaulted ceilings...creating an air of spaciousness and lightness. In one room, there are seating sections for families to gather and congregate. A big fish tank provides some color and life next to the information desk and even the chairs are cushy, big, and roomy. In the waiting area closest to the hospital entrance, the seating is more conventional...but the piece de resistance is the baby grand piano. Stately and with a black shine, it is the focal centerpiece of the room. Little did I realize the comfort it would provide me daily. Often, this is where I would retreat to write and shed my tears while listening to the classical pieces so eloquently played by the volunteer pianists.

November 13 at 6:15pm
Surgery Update

Just want to share with you an update on Mom's surgery. She is now out of surgery, in recovery, and expected to be in ICU for the next day or two. The surgery went as well as could be expected and I'll keep you updated as she progresses.

At one point during surgery, I heard an announcement on the intercom, "Paging Dr. Lerner, please call extension 2342." Then a few hours later I would hear, "Paging Dr. Edraki, please call extension 4586."

Initially, I panicked thinking something was going wrong with Mom's surgery. And maybe it was. I'll never know. But then I remembered Dr. Lerner telling me that both he and Dr. Edraki would be operating together on Mom, accompanied by a few other supporting surgeons and nurses. There was a whole team in on this one. Periodically, a nurse would come over and provide us with an update. Finally, at 6:30pm, Dr. Lerner walked into the waiting room. Smartly dressed in his scrubs with a bandana and glasses on, I saw for the first time his real work uniform. Over nine hours had passed since our last exchange, and I thought he looked a little tired but quite good for having gotten through a longer than expected surgery. Hadn't I warned him? Nothing was usual or ordinary with Mom.

We all stood up to respectfully greet Dr. Lerner and he sat down with us and proceeded to explain,

"The surgery went well, and I was successful in removing all the cancer I could see. Dolly is now in ICU, and we expect her to be here for a day or two as we manage the fluid shift."

"We did the tumor debulking, performed a hysterectomy, removed the omentum (lining of her stomach), spleen, appendix, lining of her diaphragm, and a portion of her colon (large and small intestine). Tumors were also removed from her liver and abdomen."

If there was anything else mentioned, I didn't hear

it. I could hardly keep up. While family members had a few other questions for Dr. Lerner, there was only one that I needed to ask.

Nervous, I hesitantly inquired, "Dr. Lerner, did you have to do a colostomy?" I could see my family look at me oddly with a "Why are you asking him that question?"

He looked me straight in the eyes and with a faint smile replied, "No, I did not have to do a colostomy."

With a huge sigh of relief, I smiled and graciously thanked him. It was the little secret between us, and we both knew the magnitude of what this meant. He had just earned another stripe with Mom even though she didn't know it yet.

Later that evening, Aunt Beth and I went to see Mom in the ICU.

A quiet hum of the ventilator in the quiet of the night. Unresponsive to us, her head was twitching, and it really unnerved me. She didn't look like herself and it was the worst visual I've ever had of Mom. Sometimes I wish I'd never seen her like that. But I needed to let her know we were there and that she got through it.

Thursday, November 14

This morning I went to the ICU at around 9:30am to check in on my mom and bring the nurses some goodies. I figure it can only help to "butter them up" with treats and kindness. After all, they are taking great care of Mom! Patti her primary nurse (on day shift) is great – she is a young, vibrant, little pistol and so attentive and caring. I was a bit taken aback when they asked me to wait for about 10 minutes this morning before letting me in. Going with the flow, I hung out in the waiting room until Patti showed up and said I can come visit my mom now – they had just taken her off the ventilator! Such great news! So, I'm happy to report that although Mom is still in the ICU, she is off the machine! Just going to check in on her again now for another update. Thank you all for your prayers and well wishes. And a huge thank you to all the Yountville dancers – heard you had a little "posse get together" in honor of my mom. It is all helping immensely!

Friday, November 15
Sitting in a chair at the side of her bed, I held her hand and said my prayers.

I was able to see Dr. Lerner last night and get the full update on Mom. The surgery, although extensive, went great. And although she is missing a few parts, it is nothing that we can't live without! So, Dr. Lerner certainly upheld his end of the deal and now it's up to Mom and her "Special Ops" team to keep moving in the right direction on a path to recovery.

Last night we had a bit of a cardiac scare, apparently Mom got agitated, fired one of her ICU nurses and went code blue but all is under control and Mom is stable. (Could this have been the episode in the hospital that Christine was referring to?) This morning, they got her out of bed and sitting up in a chair for a little while, too. I think she really enjoyed getting out of that bed, even if just for an hour! She had a really good morning visit with my dad. And someone from St. John Vianni Church comes each day to give a blessing and this morning Aunt Beth and I were there to share in the blessing for Mom.

This weekend the other surgeon, Dr. Edraki, will check in on Mom. So great to know that one of them is checking on her each day. Her day nurse Patti is AMAZING (as are Linda and Kim). Patti is the perfect personality to handle Mom, especially when she gets feisty. You know she's got an eye on these nurses and watching every move they make. She doesn't really tolerate ineptitude, as I'm sure you tap dancers are all too aware of! They are hoping to get her out of the ICU tomorrow, but only time will tell. Also, my brother Joe has posted the photo of all the tappers in their pink hats from Wednesday night in her room – she loves it! As I close out, I'm sitting in one of the main waiting rooms and the pianist is playing. (I wondered if anyone actually played this beautiful piece). He is absolutely wonderful. If Donna, Sheilah, Marianne, Carol, and all the Yountville tappers were here, I know you'd all be standing by his side singing away with him! Have a great day everyone and I'll be in touch.

Alone in the ICU with Mom, Dr. Edraki entered the room – he was on duty today to cover patient rounds. While I will never know if Dr. Lynn Kowalski's call spurred this act of generosity, I'll forever be grateful to him for this gracious act of kindness. We would get a 2-for-1 extended stay rate and I would also be checking in to 5 West with Mom. The doctors arranged for me to stay in the room with Mom once she got out of the ICU. I was going to be her roommate in Hell.

Saturday, November 16

Today has been a busy day and all good news to report. Mom is off oxygen (a few tubes removed!) and early this morning they had her walking the hallway. These nurses do not mess around! And then Mom spent quite a bit of time sitting up in a chair enjoying the late morning sun. If you didn't know, Saturday is "spa day" here with some great pampering! Mom's nurse today, Shaheen, is also AMAZING! She gave her a nice shampoo (the technology these days!), scalp massage, and shoulder/back massage. I asked her if she was available for house calls!

Dr. Edraki came to check on Mom today and he also confirmed how pleased he was with the surgery (he was in OR for her surgery tag-teaming with Dr. Lerner). He is also very happy with Mom's progress thus far and issued release orders to get her out of the ICU. I'm sure you can only imagine she has made it very clear to everyone that she does not want to be in this ICU room anymore. So, I just got the call at 4:30 pm that she will be moving out of the ICU and into **Room 589**. Please note that **THE NO VISITORS OR PHONE CALLS POLICY WILL CONTINUE TO BE ENFORCED UNTIL FURTHER NOTICE**. If you wish to be in contact with Mom, feel free to send a card to John Muir Medical Center in Walnut Creek – I know she'd love to hear from everyone, and it'll also give her something to do! (I think she's going stir crazy already.) All in all, everything is going great. It's just a tough, bumpy road she's traveling on now...I'm looking forward to getting her room all comfy for her and hopefully it'll bring a little more peace and tranquility to her stay here. Signing off for now – a great evening to all!

CHAPTER 8

WELCOME TO 5 WEST

Lizard Spends the Night

Fred here sending an update *(this is my brother writing under one of his nicknames)*

The Leapin' Lizard *(one of my family nicknames)* was given the green light by the physician to spend the night in the room with Mom. They have these pull-out chair gizmos that unfold into a twin-size pad of sorts. So, I'll be tip toeing around Lizann today in the event she didn't get much sleep. Gotta love that family gene of little food and little sleep. :)

Mom is miserable, but battling. As expected, the post-op pains are hitting hard and heavy. The cards, photos, and well wishes are being well received. THANK YOU! Mom reads them when she can.

Mom was moved out of the ICU yesterday afternoon (Yay!) and into a nice corner suite room looking out over Ignacio Valley Road. The full moon makes for a nice night light. But it also makes for lots of lullabies sounding throughout the hospital's intercom system. Every time a baby is born, they play a little jingle. Full moons and their gravitational pull tend to keep the labor and delivery rooms busy.

Happy Sunday morning to everyone. Say some prayers in church today and let the sun shine down upon your families with warmth and comfort. Hug your loved ones tight!

Sunday, November 17

The past 24 hours have been a bit of a roller coaster ride...some ups and some downs. Last night had some challenges and right now Mom is battling with atrial fibrillation and fluid in the lungs (pulmonary edema). They've administered some cardiac medication and Lasix to get the fluid out of her system. As you can imagine, this all seems to frustrate her a bit as a minor roadblock. And let's throw some sleep deprivation in the mix as icing on the cake. Oh, what fun!

The upside is that she took two laps "around the track" today and is clipping along at a pretty good speed! Just enough to tire her out for a follow up "nap in the chair." This evening Dr. Edraki came by to check up on Mom and I think he's already got her number! He reiterated that she needs to take it easy, relax, and not rush anything. He asked her if she was in a hurry! LOL. Another little step forward is that she can now chew gum. So, I've got her on a dose of "passion fruit" and will change it up tomorrow! Going to keep her on her toes. As my Uncle Netto used to say, "inch by inch." Signing out for tonight…

Monday, November 18

Last night was definitely a bit better, although Mom is still sorting through cardio and pulmonary issues. But the doctors are all checking on her regularly and monitoring accordingly. At 3pm today, Mom had her first confrontation with physical therapy. Laura had her doing all sorts of exercises – a little warm up before the "walking tour" and a little cool down afterwards.

Today's objective from Dr. Lerner: Walk three laps "around the track." Result: I say two times, but Mom is claiming 2.5 due to the fact that she had to walk to the gurney today (for her abdominal and chest X-rays). Not to mention that she said opening all the cards you've sent exhausted her and should count for something. So, I'll concede this round to her. I guess you could say my new nickname is "The Enforcer." A very special and heartfelt thank you to everyone who has sent cards to Mom. My dad came down this morning for a brief visit and made the postal delivery. So wonderful to see all the love and caring coming her way! She is so overwhelmed by it all and so thankful to all of you. And she is looking forward to reading all your comments on this web page, but she's not quite up to it yet. Side note: her dose of gum today was cinnamon. Figured I'd give a little something to spice her up!

To round out the busy day, this evening she had a very brief visit from Joe, Janine, Gabriella, and Dominic. It exhausted her, but she especially loved getting the latest and greatest updates from the kids! She is now resting comfortably, and I can only hope for a peaceful and restful sleepover tonight.

Tuesday, November 19
Turning A Corner

Another long and restless night for our "sleepover" yesterday evening. Add to that the "construction zone" on the wing as well. I don't know what would possess someone to be sanding down the floors from 7pm-11pm, but that's what they were doing. Along with meds, the nurses were handing out ear plugs! Not to worry – my brother came up with a brilliant solution today (yes, the sanding continues tonight, too). Mom now using his noise-canceling headphones! Even better! If you didn't know it, this Special Ops team is all about finding solutions to even the smallest of problems. Thank you, Joe!

I named this entry "Turning A Corner" because that is what I think last night and today was. We had "Monday Midnight Massage" and she got a good little scalp, shoulder, and back massage. She also read for about 30 minutes and went through the entire guestbook on this site. That tuckered her out for a little while!

Then imagine this scenario: it is 3am and Mom is wide awake – first she decides to straighten up her tray table (of course, everything needs to be in its proper place), then she decides to comb her hair and lastly, she reminds me to make sure I add water to the flowers. If that's not the Dolly we know and love, I don't know what is! I was chuckling to myself inside as I watched all this unfold. And she doesn't think she's getting any better! Lol.

This morning we woke up around 7am to the sound of that sweet lullaby – a little Scorpio baby just born! And today was a very busy day. Dr. Lerner came by for an early morning visit during our "spa day" and gave a little chuckle as Mom explained that she was getting her beauty parlor treatments. I think his response was something along the lines of that a walk around the track would be a great follow up to her spa treatment. Ha! He said everything is progressing nicely – lots of rumblings going on internally and he also gave the go ahead for a few more tubes to be removed.

Then Mom proceeds to start questioning Dr. Lerner if he'd already done surgery this morning (he had). And of course, she starts probing for more info. He had this little smirk on his face and I'm surmising that he too senses she is rounding the corner. So, after our "spa appointment" at 9am, her nurse Katie (absolutely adorable and knows how to work Mom) suggested that they follow it up with a lap around the track (just in time for the doc to see and earn her some brownie points). Even Katie received "the look" from Mom, but she handled Mom's stubborn ways brilliantly. Yes, mission accomplished as Dr. Lerner gave her a little compliment and smile.

We were off to a busy start to the day! By 10am she was already tuckered out and ready for a snooze. She then had a nice, short visit with my dad, Aunt Beth, and Uncle Keith. At 3pm, Laura was to make her PT appearance and Mom knew she was going to have to perform. So, she rested up for this one. Result: Lap 2 accomplished with a lovely warm up and cool down.

All the docs and nurses say she is doing great, and I just wish she would believe everyone! I think tomorrow is going to be a GREAT day for her and I'm looking forward to marking her one week in the hospital with lots of positive energy and love. Hoping that her discomfort continues to subside and that the love from everyone overshadows the tough moments. Signing off for tonight as I just heard another sweet lullaby...sweet dreams!

Wednesday, November 20
A Tribute to Mom
Last night was a bit restless and again at 2am we were

cleaning up and rearranging the room (or rather I was the one rearranging and following orders). Finally, a bit of REM sleep was achieved only to be woken at 7am to the sound of that sweet-sounding lullaby. Shortly thereafter there was an appearance by Dr. Devain – the cardiologist who's all heart! This guy always shows up early and catches us off guard. His update: a favorable report and looking good.

Then Dr. Lerner makes his first of two appearances to check on Mom. Of course, Mom gets the lowdown on his case load for today and begins the probe on his two scheduled surgeries. I think he's getting used to her inquisitive nature! (She even pulled a fast one on me and made Dr. Lerner wish me a happy birthday in Russian and write it on the whiteboard.) To change up the morning routine, Mom then got a foot soak and bath followed by a lap around the track. All this before 9:30am. Off to a very busy morning...by 1pm Mom has accomplished three laps around the track and, in fact, the track has been lengthened to now incorporate the hallway – I like to call it the home stretch! Great progress over yesterday in the walking department! Side note: we counted at least six Scorpio babies born today. These are my peeps!

In closing, I want to commemorate this journal entry as a "thank you tribute" to my mom. It was on this day, just a few years ago (so I say) that my mom gave me the greatest gift of all – the gift of life. How appropriate that I can share my special birthday today with her (I'm not usually with family on my birthday, so this is an extra special gift). Mom said from the minute I was born, the doctor told her I was a fighter (I was a preemie and only had a 50/50 chance of survival). Today, just a few years later (ok, 40 something), I continue to fight – not for me, but for Mom and her battle. So, today, I honor the special and amazing woman who brought me into this world and raised me with all the love, compassion, and support a daughter could ever hope for. Mom, ILYMTT! Buona notte, dorme bene e sogni d'oro!

Thursday, November 21

One thing I can say for certain is that some things with mothers never change! Last night I went to celebrate my birthday by having dinner with my brother, Joe, at the Kensington Fire Station where he was working. He made a fabulous duck dinner and I got to enjoy a relaxed and fun-filled evening with the crew. If I ever ran into a problem, these are the people I want helping me! The evening was full of laughter and crazy stories that only firefighters can tell! I'm sure you can imagine that when I wasn't back in the room at 10pm, my mom started to worry. Apparently, she was ready to call in the cavalry.

Luckily, I walked in the door right after she called Joe. I certainly don't want her blood pressure to get out of control over that and then I have to do some explaining to the docs. After all these years, nothing has changed! She's still looking out for me even when she's miserable and in the hospital. That's my mom, Dolly!

Of course, there are a few things which are fast becoming "rituals." I really need to nip this one in the bud, because sleep deprivation does not become me! Once again at 2am, Mom is awake and "kicking the covers." She's restless, so I suggest she take an early morning stroll. She actually listened to me and took my advice. So, there she was roaming the halls in the wee hours of the morning. Then out of nowhere she comments on how her staples are not in a straight line. I told her she was going to have to take that up with Dr. Lerner!

Fatigue finally set in, and she got in a few good hours of sleep. Thank goodness because I really wasn't in the mood for more organizing or room rearranging. And then again like clockwork, that cardiac doctor comes waltzing in the door at 7am! No warning at all, so there we are all disheveled and barely awake. Mom actually asked him if he had a golf game today because he came in so early! He even chuckled at that one. And as usual, Dr. Lerner followed up with his visit around 8am – scrubs on and all. Another day of surgery. After his assessment of Mom's progress (all good and moving forward) Mom, of course, proceeds to chat him up and ask him about last night (she heard him being paged throughout the evening). Pretty soon this doc is going to think she's stalking his every move!

By 9am, the revolving door of nurses and doctors coming through subsided a bit. With a bit of down time to think and plan, Mom decides she needs some air freshener for the room! And of course, the nurses delivered. As for progress, Mom has taken the next step and is now on clear liquids (although she says the Jello sucks, but the sorbet is good). Pretty soon, she'll be menu planning! But her insides are still rumbling and it's not easy going. Seems to be one thing after another. But I guess that's all part of the healing process. Side note: she did get a reprieve today on the "laps around the track." She needed today to just rest and sleep. So, this afternoon was all about cat naps. And hopefully tonight will be a peaceful sleep. On that note, signing out and wishing you all a very peaceful night's rest.

Friday, November 22

For whatever reason, it seems to be the nighttime "activities" that garner the best stories for Mom's daily updates! Perhaps it's because it's late at night, she's tired, uncomfortable, bored of being confined to that hospital bed, tired of being poked and prodded every couple of hours, and having to endure all of this without any real food consumption. That would certainly send me over the edge.

So last night at about 9:30pm, out of the blue, I get the directive to get on the phone and call my Aunt Beth (my mom's younger sister) in Santa Rosa. I was given the task to call and remind her that under no circumstances can she use paper napkins at Thanksgiving dinner (she is hosting this year). I was like, "seriously?" Yes, she was dead serious. It must have been weighing heavily on my mom's mind as she normally hosts the annual Thanksgiving soiree for our huge family get together. Obviously, there are certain standards here that need to be upheld and Mom is on it. End result: mission accomplished, and my aunt can borrow all the lincn napkins she wants from my mom!

Then from out of left field, (I guess she felt that she was on a roll, so why stop now?) Mom proceeded to tell me how she doesn't like my perfume (Dior Addict, if you must know). She said if I kept wearing it, she wouldn't let me hug her anymore. So, in the trash it went! Yep, true story. Perhaps I can ask Santa for a new perfume for Christmas that is acceptable to Mrs. Claus?

This morning like clockwork, we awoke at 6:30 am to that sweet-sounding lullaby. It really is the perfect way to get your day off to a great start! As Mom is turning that corner, she's now getting fussy – with her food, of course. She says the ginger ale doesn't taste like ginger ale and the Jello doesn't taste like Jello. I told her it's "institutional cuisine," which she obviously is not accustomed to. A little later than usual this morning, the cardiac doctor makes his rounds (guess he didn't have a round of golf today).

And this afternoon Mom had a visit with my dad, a brief visit from Fr. John for a little prayer, and then a nice nap. She knew what was coming up and had to preserve her energy. You'll all be happy to know that Mom was back out on the track with Laura her PT coach this afternoon. They did the pre-requisite warm up, a nice long lap, and a cool down. Today also marked another milestone – Mom asked for a hair dryer and her curlers! Now, that must be a good sign! I'm sure the makeup request will soon follow.

Around 5pm, Dr. Lerner made his appearance after his day of surgery. He and Mom had a great long chat (really it was her drilling him with probing questions) and it was nice to just sit back and observe their interaction. At one point though, I thought Mom was going to ruin the moment. She asked him why her staples weren't in a straight line. Without missing a beat, he answered, "Just tilt your head when you're looking at them." Ha! We were totally cracking up!

Suffice to say, today was a better day than yesterday and Mom also got the "go ahead" to have solid food. And I'm sure that mashed potatoes will be high on her wish list! So, another day of progress has been made and I suspect that we only have a few more days here before we can escape! I couldn't ask for anything better from today. Although we are enjoying our "sleepover," we are both looking forward to getting back to "home sweet home." On that note, may you all enjoy the comforts of your own home tonight...signing out and wishing all a peaceful night's sleep.

Saturday, November 23

Today was a day all about relaxation for Mom. There seems to be much more quiet and calm on 5 West now. Perhaps it's because there are no bells or whistles constantly beeping and going off in her room. With Mom off all machines now (yay!), the silence is truly golden! Last night was actually quite uneventful – no crazy talk, organizing, or rearranging. Although at some ungodly hour she did threaten that if I didn't change the water in the flowers, she was going to make a call to Sylvie (my friend in Canada) and anyone else who sent flowers! Suffice it to say, all the flowers have clean, fresh, clear water now.

And we skipped the nighttime stroll because she just wasn't up to it. Not to worry, I know I'll get her lap in around that track at some point! Dr. Lerner paid us a visit early this morning (after already completing one surgery) and the topic of "release" came up. We are looking at Monday for a possible escape!

I knew what was coming…planning and scheming for the return home. Where will Mom sleep? What do we need? So, at 9am the list gets started. I'm sure it'll be a work in progress, and I can only hope that she won't have me working on this at 2am!

Moving on, the late morning consisted of a brief visit by my dad, Aunt Beth, and Uncle Keith. I was "off duty" for a couple hours and had gone out to San Ramon to watch my nephew play a baseball game. Ok, I digress momentarily as I brag for a minute – my nephew, Dom, was invited to play with this team of high school kids from all throughout the area. He was one of four eighth graders invited to participate, and he did great! What an amazing experience for him and a great introduction and leap to the next level of baseball. Yes, I was a proud aunt this afternoon!

After his game, Dom and I formulated a game plan to surprise my mom. Our strategy consisted of first going to the grocery store to buy her real ginger ale (Canada Dry, of course!) and Jello pudding. We then had to create a little diversion to smuggle the goods "in house." I don't know what the rules are on that, but neither of us wanted to get caught and find out. Mission accomplished and we strolled right through the 5 West Wing. Dom was still in his uniform and greeted my mom with a huge smile and hug. And I know that today, Dom was the highlight of my mom's day! He recounted for her the game and what it was like to play with all these older and more experienced high school kids. It was priceless, quality time spent between a grandmother and her grandson. A memory that will last forever.

Later this evening, Mom decided it was time to hit the track! We finally figured out that if you go later in the evening, you miss the "rush hour traffic" and you can have the home stretch all to yourself! So, at 8:30 pm, we start with a little warm-up (you all know how important that is.)

So, I say, "Let's start with some ankle mobility..." and before I know it, Mom is sitting on the side of the bed doing shuffle ball change combinations with her feet. I did a double take and started laughing, as I mustered a little "What was that?" We both had a good laugh with that for a minute.

We finally depart the room and go for our little evening stroll. It's open highway and Mom is clipping along at a pretty good pace with her walker. We make a few stops along the way looking at the various boards, then make our way back. We get back to the room to retire for the evening and as I glance over at Mom to ask a question, I see that she's fast asleep. That's my signal and signing off for tonight... and wishing you all a peaceful sleep, too.

Sunday, November 24
Untitled By Joe Grupalo
Hats off to the Lizard. Always working, always shar-

ing. Between taking notes during doctors' visits, typing daily blogs, sparring with Mom to keep moving, supporting Mom to keep her spirits high, and motivating her for more shuffle ball changes – she still finds time to go to the ball park, visit the firehouse, and share dinners with her little bro's family.

Long nights and little sleep shows in her eyes, but not in her endless smiles. Angels are everywhere in Walnut Creek. Thanks for all you're doing for Mom and the family. The Leapin' Lizard Lives!

Sunday, November 24

Today was another interesting day...not so much with what Mom did, but by the people we are surrounded by on 5 West. I'll get to that a little later. First, a little recap from last night's sleepover. The door continues to revolve on a regular basis with nurses coming in to poke and prod. At one point, Mom and I were wide awake and around 1:30am she looks at me and asks, "When will we get a good night's sleep?" I surmise that it probably won't be until we are home in our own beds...soon, very soon.

I could tell that when she woke up this morning, she was a bit cranky (to be expected). But she added fuel to the fire when she got up to go to the bathroom and decided to stop in front of the mirror.

She took one look in the mirror and exclaimed, "Oh my God!"

I responded, "I told you not to look in the mirror!"

(Which I had been telling her repeatedly.)

I've been looking in it each morning and it's just not a pretty picture right now (and I haven't even had surgery). But I'm going to chalk it up to "bad fluorescent lighting" and leave it at that.

Dr. Lerner made his appearance around 9am this morning and I'm happy to report that TUESDAY will be our escape – we'll be flying this coop! I think the extra day will be great for Mom – she needs one more heart test tomorrow and we can get her all primped and pretty for the return home.

So, back to the doc. As we were chatting away, I knew it was just a matter of time before Mom made it all personal again. She told him that she'd been doing some thinking…see, we discovered that he's going to get married in Calistoga next year and that it'll be a Russian-Jewish wedding. Well, with all the free time on Mom's hands, I should have known… she's already planning this guy's wedding for him! She offered up her ideas on wedding planning and recounted for him how her friend Sheilah was married at their home in Yountville. Mom advised him to incorporate all the Jewish traditions and even asked about the music selections. This poor guy! I told Dr. Lerner to tread cautiously with Mom in releasing wedding information, as she could end up being a wedding crasher!

By 10am, we had taken a lap around the track

and Mom was ready for some rest. It's just so hard when you can't sleep at night, so I'm just encouraging her to take the little cat naps whenever she can. The afternoon was very uneventful aside from the revolving door of nurses to administer shots, check levels, etc. We took an afternoon stroll and hit the home stretch in full stride and then followed it up with a great nap.

We were soon chatting with Monica, Mom's RN today, and she asked us if we'd seen the "naked man" a few doors down. We had seen a rather large man in the room but hadn't really paid too much attention. He is our "neighbor" two doors down and is quite a large man – who is naked in his room. Apparently, he doesn't like to wear clothes...and supposedly he's partial to sprawling out in certain positions in bed, too (so says the nurse). Mom and I decide that we'll try to catch a glance and check this out (but we don't really want to see anything!).

This evening we had dinner together and Mom is starting to eat a bit more. Yes, she had mashed potatoes and gravy tonight with a little piece of chicken!

Then around 7:30 pm, we decide to take another evening stroll. This is great progress, as we are up to three laps today! And now is the perfect time to do some recon on the naked man next door. As we exit the room and start our little shuffle down the hall, we're battling a bit of rush hour traffic. They weren't kidding. You have to pick a lane and stay there! We're disappointed to find out that naked man has escaped. Checked out.

But before you know it, we pass another "walker" down the hallway and notice something strange. She appears to be walking with her husband, but another man is trailing her. We don't think much of it, except that I had mentioned to Mom yesterday that I thought there was a bodyguard outside of a room (near the main nurse's station). As we are coming down the home stretch, we pass them again (give a nod and smile) and then we both catch it this time – the woman is in chains! She is pushing her walker, trailing with the IVs, and chains clanking at her ankles. I look up at the guy who is following and see "prison guard" embroidered on his sleeve. OMG, we both look at each other with eyes open wide and decide to pick up our pace a little bit and get back to our room.

So now I've got a new mission and am trying to do some recon to find out who this woman is from the jail. But I am not getting anywhere. They are all pretty tight-lipped. I've even bribed them with some Trader Joe's "dunkers" – biscuits with chocolate. But no luck yet. Not to worry...I'm still on it and tomorrow is another day. Just need to find the right "asset" to work with.

So, a bit of an exciting day here on 5 West. Funny how the littlest things can provide such intrigue and entertainment. That's all for now and signing off for tonight…Mom is sound asleep and resting comfortably. Wishing you all a wonderful and peaceful sleep!

Monday, November 25
Last Night on 5 West

I knew today was going to be off to a rocky start when I woke up to the sound of "tray organizing." I figured that "Cranky Pants" Mom was restless again and knew I had to nip this in the bud right away. Disheveled and with an early morning smile, I asked Mom if she was going to need an attitude adjustment today. No answer, but I did get a little smirk. And that was fine by me. Point made and taken.

The early morning was quiet and peaceful as Mom tried to catch up on some sleep. Then Dr. Lerner dropped by around 9:30am (late for him – but we figured he'd already done at least one surgery this morning as he was in his scrubs) for the check-in, and we discussed a few concerns (or rather I did).

Biggest issue today: Mom has no appetite! That is so NOT a Sladek/Grupalo trait! Something is definitely out of sorts! Well, wait until you hear this one – it's about to get really good. Dr. Lerner, leaning against the wall with his arms crossed, offers up a solution – he says Mom can take Marinol, and we sort of look at each other and then back at the doctor. We had no idea what that was. He said she can have marijuana! So, there's Mom – getting high on marijuana today to get her appetite back. She gets to "light up" twice a day! Ha! One more "hit" coming tonight...FYI, Mom wanted me to make sure I point this out to Gretchen, Randi, and Marianne! Mom says you are the "hippie" girls and will appreciate this. So, I haven't noticed any odd behavior yet, but I think I'm going to try and get her to take to the highway for a stroll and see what happens. This could get really good...and especially when we come round the corner to the jailbird's room.

Yes, I've done my recon and have figured out that our "inmate" is in Room 581. She is literally sequestered in that room all day (with the prison guard) and only gets to come out for one walk (usually in the evening). I also figured out that she's in the federal prison, but I can't get any info as to what she's in for. One of the other nurses (her identity will remain undisclosed) tried to find out and they wouldn't give up any information. I think only the charge nurse is "in the know."

We also discovered that Cynthia M. (Mom's RN today) is from Lima, Peru and she is FABULOUS! I had a long chat with her about Peru and Cynthia was even able to convince Mom to let her remove the staples tonight. Otherwise, Mom was threatened with the possibility that a student nurse would show up tomorrow morning to do the job. Mom was having none of that.

So, the magic number: 45 staples removed. That

is the new removal record, even for Cynthia (which beats her previous record of 35). Cynthia also shared with us (in confidence) that she is eight weeks pregnant! So, exciting for her and her husband… and this will be their third child. It is all hush-hush and on the down low right now, but we are in the know. What a great Christmas present for her family (when she'll unveil the surprise).

The other great news is that by 9pm Mom hit her milestone achievement: four laps around the track! I was seriously on a mission to achieve our goal of four laps before our escape. Mom still uses the walker, but she's clipping along at a good pace. Of course, we slow upon approaching Room 581 and I strain to hear anything I can, but no deal. The door is closed and not a peep can be heard. The highway stroll was quite uneventful and very quiet. We did pass a poster on the wall about "Attitude" and I made Mom listen to me read part of it. In my mind, it's all part of the healing process – you really have to have the right attitude. Point made again and taken.

So, tonight is our last night on 5 West. It's been such an interesting journey here (definitely a roller coaster ride) and Mom has come so far. It's hard to believe we've been here almost two weeks.

I know many of you wanted to come and visit Mom in the hospital and she truly appreciates you honoring her wish for no visitors. I hope you understand that it's because she is so exhausted and just doesn't have the energy to talk or to even listen at times. I know that in time, she'll reach out to all of you and will eventually be up for little visits. And there's nothing I would rather see than Mom surrounded by her loving friends and family in the comfort of her own home. Tomorrow we are coming home, to the place that holds such a special place in her heart – one of peace, tranquility, and filled with endless love. And I must admit, for purely selfish reasons, I can't wait to sleep in a real bed again!

So, here's to our last night on 5 West. And for this last night, I want to close out by honoring all the doctors and nurses who have given Mom such brilliant care these past two weeks: Dr. Lerner and Dr. Edraki (amazing and gifted surgeons); Dr. Devain (cardiologist); Dr. Gill (anesthesiologist); Margaret in pre-op; Sue in the OR; and Patti, Linda, and Shaheen (her brilliant and amazing RNs in ICU). And to all the RNs and RNAs of 5 West – thank you for getting Mom back on her feet and ultimately home: Charlotte (so helpful to Mom in her first two nights on 5 West), Christine, Janus, Janet, Jenny, Katie (worked wonders in getting Mom to walk), Ebony, Dennis, Mercy, Ochi, Hiwot (so sweet with her incredible desire to help Mom whenever needed), Priscilla, Anne, Delia, Nicole, Monica, and to her last two nurses who truly had a positive impact and made a lasting impression on Mom – Cynthia M. (from Peru) and Cynthia N. (from The Philippines). The care you give is remarkable and truly memorable. And I hope you know that you've made a difference in our family's life. Thank you from the bottom of my heart! God bless and good night.

CHAPTER 9

A NEW SET OF HURDLES

Wednesday, November 27
Home Sweet Home

We are finally home, but it wasn't an easy journey getting here. Our last night on 5 West was as good as we could hope for – quite uneventful with just the usual comings and goings by the nurses. No crazy late-night excursion from the lady in chains and the naked man is gone. Mom's vitals are all good, consistent, and on track. And yesterday morning was great for Mom to get in her first shower (plus a shampoo and a style). Although I must admit, I'm really not a good stylist, so the style was a little lacking. But I gave it a valiant effort. I guess I should say it was more like a shampoo and an attempted blow out. And again, I reminded Mom NOT to look in the mirror! (Of course, she did). Even so, it was all good prep for the arrival home.

We left the hospital around 11am yesterday and Joe was a tremendous help to come over to the hospital after he got off work at the fire station to help us load up the car. You would have thought we were going on a cross country trip with all the bags we had! We were definitely leaving with more than we came with. And of course, the nurses were great and let us stockpile a few goodies to take home. As for the car ride home, it was long and tough for Mom with all the motion. One good thing I can say is that she took a fabulous nap once she got settled in. It was a good three-hour nap, uninterrupted. Now, that was a first! The quiet, peacefulness, and comfort of being in your own home is definitely something to be thankful for.

Being home, however, we are faced with a whole new set of hurdles to tackle. It's a bit trying to figure out all the meds and how Mom reacts to them (some more quickly than others). As Dr. Lerner said, it'll take some time to figure out the right balance. So, I must confess we are a bit off kilter at the moment. Ironically enough, I never thought I would be the one to be administering pot to my mom! Does that make me a legalized drug dealer? Hmm...Yes, the pot continues – as she has a one-month prescription. And FYI, that stuff is really expensive (even with insurance). When the pharmacist told me the price, I was so tempted to just get her a few joints, call it a day, and save the money! But then I thought that may cause more problems – especially if I got caught and hauled off to the Napa Jail! It's trial and error with food and I'm hoping the pot kicks in soon! We need to get her energy up.

Today, while everyone else was out buying ingredients to make their Thanksgiving dinners for tomorrow – turkey, stuffing, gravy, sweet potatoes, and pumpkin pie – I was buying Jello, pudding, apple sauce, and mashed potatoes. Those are the few things that she can tolerate right now. I'm sure the grocery checkers thought I was off my rocker! Not to worry, I will try to concoct some sort of Thanksgiving dinner for her and my dad. It might not be our "traditional" fare – but, hey, rules are meant to be broken, right?

Most important to me is that Mom is home and will be with family tomorrow. I know she is feeling really lousy right now –but I'm hoping that in the end, she'll look back on the day with contentment – to be home for Thanksgiving with her family, on this very special holiday that is one of her favorites!

I will also remind her (in case she cops an attitude) that we have so, so much to be thankful for! She has gotten past the surgery with the best doctors and nurses, and she is now home and "on the road" (albeit a slow one) to recovery. Not to mention that when she is home, she is certainly not alone (although I suspect that she yearns for some alone time away from us all!). I think of all the people who are in the hospital or those who are home, but all alone. I count my blessings for the special family we have. And Mom is certainly blessed to have all the wonderful friends that she does (and across so many miles)! Of course, I will remind her of all this tomorrow.

So, a big "thank you" to all of Mom's friends and family – especially her siblings: Beth, Bunny, and Chuck. THANK YOU for blessing her life with your presence and for your continued outpouring of love and support! I can't wait for her to feel better to read all your wonderful, loving, and thoughtful messages. Oh, and not to worry – I'll keep up with the journal, so you are updated on Mom's progress. I'm not sure it'll be as frequent or as colorful as 5 West with all the "inmates," but I promise you'll be kept in the loop on how things are going and when she'll be up for phone calls or visits. For now, it's all about quiet and rest for Mom. My goal: to get her in her "recovery groove."

So, as I sign off, here's my wish for all – take a good look at who you are with tomorrow as you celebrate Thanksgiving. Look them in the eyes, give them a big hug and a kiss, and thank them for their presence in your life. Here's wishing you and your families a very special and wonderful Thanksgiving tomorrow. Yes, we really do have so much to be thankful for!

Wednesday, December 4
Three Weeks Post Surgery

Hi all, I'm back to report on Mom's progress! Yes, I've received a few "we need an update" emails as a gentle reminder to keep you all in the loop. You all know who you are! Apologies, as I've been just a bit overwhelmed of late and frankly not in the mood to write. But I think I've turned my corner. Ha!

Well, it is so hard to believe that today marks the three-week anniversary of Mom's invasive surgery. It's hard to believe it's been that long already. And while I wish I could report that all is great and she's making a speedy recovery, the reality is that this surgery really did a number on her. Coming home a week ago certainly had its challenges and there aren't any comforting, kind, and smart nurses around to gently encourage Mom to walk, eat, etc. It's just me – "the enforcer" – and let's just say, I'm sure she is a bit tired of my commentary.

The good news is that she is up and doing so much more. It's all in the little things (as I keep saying) – she's walking more and more (and even without a walker), she's "organizing" now during the daytime (thank goodness, as it now gives me a reprieve in the wee hours of the morning!), watering all her flowers and plants inside, going through all her cards, etc. There are lots of little busy things for her to do – which may exhaust her, but all in a good way.

Yesterday was such a special day. Mom had just taken a really nice shower and was finally able to put some really comfy clothes on (a first!). Then, we came out to the living room and noticed that a fire had been built. It was so nice, but it caught us off guard as that's not really something my dad would have done on a Tuesday morning. And who appears out of the blue? Joe! After enjoying one of my home-made healthy bran muffins, Mom had mentioned that next time she'd like some pancakes! Ugh.

Perfect timing, as Joe then comes walking through the door with a box of Bisquick ready to whip up some pancakes for Mom. How could he have possibly known that? I hadn't said a word. He said it's a Sladek gene! They are so cut from the same cloth, and he always seems to know what she needs. Suffice it to say, she indulged in a nice, hot pancake right off the griddle! Joe had gotten off work and ventured up to Yountville unbeknownst to us (he has a habit of making little surprise visits). I had sent him a text SOS that I thought Mom needed a "change of scenery." Joe always provides such great mojo and is a great "pick me up" for Mom. And true to form, he was exactly what she needed! So, her day got off to a great start.

Side note: I must say that I'm a bit disappointed

in the "pot pills." They don't seem to be helping that much and I am seriously considering hitting Randi up for some "brownies" (she has a "source" and knows where to get them).

Another side note: I haven't said too much to Mom, but I'm now thinking about her strategy and plan of action for the "post-surgery" recovery. Soon, we're going to have to have some tough conversations. Does Mom want to do chemo? (She's supposed to start that in about three weeks.) Are there alternative options to consider? Would Mom consider them? I'm definitely an East meets West girl when it comes to mind, body, and spirit. Perhaps it's a generational thing, but I'm pretty open-minded to alternative medicine and think it's worth exploring.

So, as all this is weighing on my mind, who do I run into the other day? I see Jaime at Whole Foods! Exactly the person I wanted to chat with to get more information on her cancer treatments, etc. It was so great to see her and chat for a few minutes. And we'll be meeting up on Thursday for a little get together!

To conclude, all in all Mom is doing great. She's walking over to the cottage, getting around more, and slowly but surely getting back to doing little things that we all take for granted. I see this as progress and moving forward...just a little slower than I know she would like. Ok, gotta run now...Mom is up and wanting some breakfast! I'm sure I'll be making a pancake...

Sunday, December 8
'Tis the Season

So, we're now in December and it all seems like such a blur that the holiday season is already here. And we're not ready! This week was spent trying to get Mom up a bit more (still slow going) and finding a way to get her in the holiday spirit. Not much spirit around here these days, but we are all trying.

She had a spa day this week, which was great – but is always exhausting. Next time I'm going for the curlers to do her hair, as my styling is still less than desirable. The appetite and food consumption seems to come and go. She did ask for a sandwich last week, so that's something new! I've been able to make some really healthy meals that agree with her, which is another good sign.

We also had our first car ride to Napa (as she's in Mrs. Claus mode!). And as her primary elf, I had duties to fulfill. Suffice to say, I think it was great to get her out of the house for a few minutes – although it was tiring for her. Progress comes and goes in the sleep department, too. She actually slept for seven hours on Friday night, which was great but not consistent yet.

Other good news is that Mom has pretty much ditched the walker and is relying on her own two feet to shuffle around! She bundles up in this cold weather and my dad takes her on walks over to the cottage and to the barn. We've got a new training circuit going!

I've got her doing some light reading and am administering a little "homework" on some of the research I've been doing. She needs to be in the loop and I'm providing all the options and resources I can. At the end of the day though, it's her life and these need to be her decisions.

We've been talking about "what's next," and it's definitely got her wheels in motion. Needless to say, we'll have lots of questions for the doc on Thursday when we see him for her follow up appointment. And Mom is being proactive in the next steps of her care, which is such an important factor in moving forward both physically and mentally. I am really so proud of her for this!

So, let's circle back to the holiday spirit for a minute. Now, while I'm a real traditionalist when it comes to Christmas, I broke my rule on the Christmas tree. I ventured upstairs to the attic (with some help from Joe) and we brought down the fake tree (ugh!) – which was already adorned with lights and ornaments. All we had to do was remove the protective cover and plug it in. And voilà, our tree was lighting up the living room and administering a little holiday cheer! I was surprised at how quickly

I caved in and while it's not my style, I know that it's bringing great joy to Mom. I think the branches need to be straightened out a bit, and I'll doctor it up with a tree skirt (if I can find it) and a few little goodies for under the tree (I'm thinking pot brownies might be a strong contender.)

In closing, I'm hopeful that we'll (ok, I guess it's really me) be able to bring some Christmas cheer home for Mom. Yes, it'll be a very different Christmas this year – but it can still be fun and bring much joy, love, and peace to all of our hearts. My goal is to ensure that the next couple of weeks will get her in the holiday spirit and that she'll find the joy that each day brings. Happy Holidays to all!

Sunday, December 15
A Week of Progress

Just wanted to touch base and give you all an update from this past week, which I might add was very, very busy! I think that's a good sign because the more Mom is up and around, the more she's got me on my toes, running around too.

The week started off with another surprise visit from Joe on Monday morning. He had gotten off work and switched to his moonlighting job as "Mom's personal chef" whipping up our grandmother Nonni's famed Risotto (a favorite of ours). He had also received three fresh (yes, still alive and pinching), Dungeness crabs from one of his work colleagues. "Sebastian and Co" were alive and well (for a short time!), lounging in our kitchen sink. Suffice to say, we had a great dinner that day!

Other weekly activities included watering the plants – yes, that is all Mom now; it's a good little project for her to manage – as well as getting that Christmas tree sorted out. Mission accomplished. I couldn't find the actual tree skirt, so I decided to get creative and improvise...she really does have a lot of tablecloths (and yes, all fabric ones to match her cloth napkins!). Side note for those of you who want to know, YES, Aunt Beth did in fact use cloth napkins for Thanksgiving! So, we have a lovely festive red tablecloth serving as our tree skirt. And the tree branches have been straightened out, with the ornaments now hanging vertically. When Mom sits in the living room, her chair is right by the tree – so at least I know she can enjoy the spirit of the holidays with this little sort-of decked out tree.

The real big event of the week was Mom's follow up appointment with Dr. Lerner on Thursday afternoon. This was her first time being in a car for a good hour's drive, so we weren't sure how it'd go. She did great and only felt a little queasy on the ride home (but then again, that is a Sladek gene in full swing). Now, the appointment with the doc – well, that one is definitely for the journal. I tell you; I couldn't make this stuff up!

So, we arrive at our appointment and are seated

in the waiting room. At that moment, there are only two other patients waiting. But of course, it would be our luck to be stuck waiting with the "chatty Cathy." No sooner are we getting comfortable in our chairs do we realize that this woman is literally talking non-stop, and not in a faint little whisper. She's talking to anyone who will listen to her. Now, Mom and I each came prepared with reading material for any "down time" we might incur and we can't even concentrate on what we're reading. There is nowhere to escape to.

She is a single mother of four boys and is having a bad hair day (she says her hair is now all frizzy from her last round of chemo), is having difficulty with her eyes and they are all dry because of her meds, and her jeans are too tight...so she's really uncomfortable. And then she really starts in because she now has an audience of three plus the staff. She is going on about her sex life and how she really used to like it, but now she's just not really turned on by it all. And she thinks it is partly due to the vaginal corrective surgery that she had. Oh, why didn't I bring my iPod with me to this appointment? Thank goodness we didn't have to hear what came next because Jackie, the nurse, called her in.

Shortly thereafter, we get called in. So, the doc comes in and the first thing he says is, "I see you've met my colorful patient."

The recap from Mom's visit with Dr. Lerner is all positive. Everything is working and functioning properly, and her recovery is on track. The only area of improvement on this "report card" was that he feels Mom should be stronger. Hopefully, this will improve as we have changed it up a bit with her pot pills. She's increased her dose (I swear they aren't really working) and we'll give that a shot. If it still isn't helping, I've got the green light to hit the streets of Berkeley! (Yes, we actually have a prescription to visit the dispensary.) Her choice: a joint or a brownie. Knowing Mom, if I were a betting woman (which I'm not – even after living in Las Vegas) – I'd put all my money on her going for the brownie! Stay tuned for if that comes to fruition.

Oh, and then, somewhere in the middle of the consultation with Dr. Lerner sitting and facing us both, Mom looks down. Then she looks up at him and with a little smile on her face says, "Hey, we have the same shoes." And they did! They had the same tennis shoes on.

We spent quite a bit of time discussing the "next step" with chemo, etc. I was prepared and came with my binder and list of questions (I'm sure he's used to it by now). I must commend this doc, as he spent so much time with us and answered all our questions and really wants to make sure Mom keeps progressing and moving forward. We know where he stands on what he would like to see Mom do – but I must admit, he does seem open-minded. He gave us the green light to have our consultation with the integrative medical oncologist and asked that I keep in touch with how it all transpires and what we find out.

Then to wrap up her visit, I'm sure you know what's coming. She just couldn't let it go. In true Dolly fashion she starts in with, "So Dr. Lerner, how are the wedding plans coming along?"

He gives a little laugh and starts chatting with Mom.

Then she really goes in for the kill and asks, "So, how did you propose?"

I was a bit surprised that she'd go this far, but then he told us – and yes, it was in Napa! So, all in all, a very good report and visit with the doc.

Then on Friday, we had errands to do...follow up lab work and chest X-ray...and then ended it on a good note with Mom getting her hair done. I knew that would make her feel a little better! (It always works for me.) The best part – it was the first day I saw her put on lipstick! A great sign! Napa being small town USA that it is, we run into Dar at the salon who was waltzing in for her blowout. So nice for Mom to get to chat with her for a few minutes!

The big party was at Connie's last Friday night and just so you all know, Mom really would have liked to have been there with everyone! After the salon, we dropped off the gifts at Connie's house and then Mom went home to relax and recover. It was a very long day for her!

And today begins a new week and the adventure continues...Mom and I are driving to Reno this afternoon for her consultation with Dr. James Forsythe tomorrow morning at the Century Wellness Center. After all my research and findings, this is an interesting and different approach, one I believe worth exploring.

So, we're packing it up today and taking a girls' road trip...our consultation tomorrow will be with two to doctors (including Dr. Forsythe) and will last about four to five hours. Depending on how Mom feels, we'll drive back home Monday afternoon or Tuesday morning. So, I must sign off now and get ready to pack it up and get on the road. And I'll be in touch later in the week with more updates. But in the meantime, Happy Trails!

Sunday, December 25
Joyeux Noël and Merry Christmas
I realize that there's been no update for over a week or so, but it's only because I've been so so busy! It's Christmas morning and the perfect time for a little gift-giving to all of you – a little update on how Mom is doing. On December 15, Mom and I drove to Reno and it was the perfect day for a scenic ride through

Tahoe – a dusting of snow on the hills and trees providing a little "wintery white wonderland" for us to enjoy (and thanks Leah Rae for the Christmas CD!). Although in retrospect, I must admit that I don't think Mom was really up for this little adventure. However, she did great on the ride up and back – which surprised us both.

We stayed at GSR (Grand Sierra Resort), as it's where I would always stay when up there for work. And I know the area pretty well, so it was easy for us to get around and there was no stress. We got checked in and then after we had a little dinner, I figured Mom certainly deserved a reward for her efforts...so she got about 15 minutes of "play time" on the slots! It's the least I could do!

On Monday, we met with Dr. Forsythe and his team and Mom heard firsthand about his methodology and approach to treating cancer, etc. It was a day of "information overload" for Mom, but as I always say "knowledge is power" – just increasing her "arsenal" to determine best course of treatment for her and her situation. They did some bloodwork and we're now just waiting to get those results. Mom also has a appointment on Tuesday with Dr. Dugan, a traditional oncologist here in Napa. This past week was a bit of a roller coaster – a few ups and downs, as to be expected. But I genuinely think she's getting a little stronger. It's just a very slow process for her and perhaps her body is in a bit of a revolt right now and just not wanting to cooperate. She did venture out a bit more with my dad for some walks and even a drive or two in the valley. I think it's important to get her out of the house and enjoying the scenery, especially in this unseasonable warm weather (it's like Vegas – mid to high 60s, clear blue skies, and not a cloud in sight!).

On Monday, I received a call from Dr. Lerner who was just checking in to see how Mom was doing. We finally connected yesterday and as I filled him on her progress (and our trip to Reno), he discussed some ideas and thoughts and made recommendations that we can also take to Dr. Dugan for further discussion on next steps. Unbeknownst to Dr. Lerner, what a great Christmas gift he just gave to me. And all with a simple phone call. He's going on vacation next week, so we'll undoubtedly have to make some decisions without his input – but he's assured me that we can always amend and adjust depending on how Mom responds. He also asked that I let him and his office know the course of treatment we decide to start with and then he'll touch base when he gets back.

Yesterday being Christmas Eve was such a very special day for our family. Although a tough day for Mom, she was a trouper and joined us for an afternoon of great family time! Joe, Janine, Gab, and Dom came up (along with Cinca and Buster, the yellow Labs) along with my Aunt Beth, Uncle Keith, and my cousin Scott. We decided to do an early dinner (at around 1:30pm) for Mom and I had set up the dining table. While it wasn't Mom's usual decked-out elegant holiday affair, it was perfect (in my eyes). And yes, I used cloth napkins, too!

Our "dinner," however, wasn't our traditional Christmas fare either. I decided we were going "French" – and I made Julia Child's "Coq Au Vin" (I've always wanted to make this) along with one of Barefoot Contessa's French "Vegetable Tian" dishes. I was a bit worried about my chicken dish, as Mom didn't want me to light the place on fire (one step in the production requires you to light the cognac on fire to burn off the alcohol). So, I didn't do it (and then worried the dish wouldn't turn out right). And luckily my cousin Scott, who is an amazing cook (he really should be a chef), helped me with my sauce (it just needed a little thickening). Oh, yes, and we splurged on French bread from Bouchon Bakery. For dessert, I made a French apple cake (no sugar!) and served it with vanilla ice cream (to hide the aesthetic imperfections of my dessert). The best part was that Mom (and Uncle Keith, who is diabetic), could enjoy all this food (sans the ice cream!). And "where is the wine?" you might be asking....my dad pulled out a bottle of Perrier-Jouet Fleur Champagne to start... and then dug into his little collection to surprise us with a bottle of Opus One 1996 for all to enjoy (yes, we properly decanted it first).

While this wasn't our traditional Christmas gathering, it was a new first – and a very special time. Side note: I really missed my grandmother Nonni not being there with us, but I like to think that she was watching over and guiding me in the kitchen.

May the memories of Christmas this year bring much joy and peace to all of you...I know it did for me and my family! Wishing you all a very Joyeux Noël (that's French for "Merry Christmas")!

Sunday, December 25
A Surprise Visit from Mrs. Claus
Hi to all – FYI, Mom has just hijacked my computer...

Merry Christmas to each of you! Just said to Lizann that it's time for me to send out a little note, so I'm using a laptop for the first time. Many thanks for all the good wishes, prayers, and special remembrances you have sent to me and my family during this time. It really helped brighten up the day!

Love and deep gratitude for your friendship and continued prayers,
Dolly

Wednesday, January 1, 2014
Happy New Year
Well, I must confess that I am glad to be out of 2013 and into the New Year. It's been a rather challenging one to say the least, especially the last couple of months. But during all difficult times, that is when

you get your "Special Ops" team in place and rally. So, that is what our family has done. I won't say it's been easy – I've certainly lost my patience on a few occasions (unfortunately, patience is not one of my virtues) and it's been a real test to be an adult living with your parents again. Never thought I'd see that day...but here we are.

The Christmas tree is still up and brings Mom great joy. She has definitely gotten stronger this past week and I can even hear it in her voice. We haven't done too much or ventured too far outside of the house this week, but yesterday was a big day. Yes, it was New Year's Eve, but Mom and I had her appointment with Dr. Dugan (the oncologist in Napa). We were also accompanied by a very dear and special friend (you know who you are!), who was there to lend her amazing support. For the first time, I saw Mom put on full makeup (not just lipstick), do her hair, and even use her curlers! She looked awesome! I actually felt a little subpar when I walked out of the house.

So, off we go to another doctor's office near Queen of the Valley Hospital in Napa. I could tell right away that Mom was in her comfort zone – with this doctor (whom many of you in Napa know from your own personal experience) as well as the fact that the office is right next to the hospital. Mom asked a lot of questions, was engaged, and took ownership of her journey.

She is working out her "road map" and it'll be on her terms; she's opting to go with the traditional chemo, which will start in the next week or so. Of course, we discussed the side effects of these drugs and I think they just suck big time. Just sayin'. It's so hard to believe that she's going to lose all her hair (not sure why that bothers me so much, but it does), have nausea (they say there are good meds for that, so we'll just have to see), and the other drug causes neuropathy (nerve pain in your hands and feet). I guess it is what it is, and I will just leave it at that.

The doc gave her a "to do" list, so we started yesterday by checking the boxes. First up was a blood test – to check her CA-125 and HE-4 markers. So, there we were in the lab at 5:30pm on New Year's Eve. Not exactly where we were wanting to be. Box checked. Done. Next up will be for Mom to do a little outpatient procedure to insert a port (for the chemo) as well as get a post-op baseline CT scan. And lastly, she has to attend a chemo seminar (not sure what that is all about, but hopefully it doesn't send her running for the hills). Overall, it was a very productive appointment and I'm guessing it's given her some relief of the anxiety of the "unknown" – but at least she now has a plan. Mom's test results will determine what chemo treatment to start with.

Today we begin the New Year and Mom suggested that we get out of the house (oh, she is finally listening to me!)...and go to the movies! What fun! This morning I made a little brunch – mushroom and asparagus quiche and then we hit the road and went to the movies to see "Saving Mr. Banks." What a great movie by the way – I just love Emma Thompson! I even let Mom splurge on her "diet" and against my better judgment let her have some popcorn (yes, even with a little butter). I must say she's been great with following my "diet" protocol and I think it's helping. She seems to feel good and eating better. It's particularly special with today being the first day of the New Year – to me, looking ahead is what the New Year is all about.

And while I certainly appreciate the past, my wish is for Mom to embrace the present and be fully focused on her future. May we all look to the New Year with optimism, encouragement, love, and joy that the future brings. Happy New Year!

January 13, 2014
Out and About

I realize that it's been over a week and not a peep from me with an update. You probably know what that means – Mom is keeping me very busy and on my toes. Here's a little recap of the past two weeks on Mom's activities and what she's been up to.

One good thing is that Mom seems to finally be listening to me! On January 2, she got a call that a few of her Napa friends (Connie, JoAnn, Mayra, and Andrea) were going to be "doing lunch" nearby and wanted to know if they could come and kidnap her for a little "outing." At first, she said "no" – but then she remembered what I've been preaching and changed her mind. Before she could even put her lipstick on, the girls were at the front door! It was so great for Mom to get out with her friends and this is exactly what "taking back your life" entails (to me at least) – doing the things you love (no matter how big or small) with the people you love the most. Just so happy to know that my "sermons" are getting through!

Then, on January 3, my Aunt Beth came over to help Mom start "Project Clear the Clutter." I'll reserve my many comments on this topic, but will just say that it's nice to see some inroads being made in this department. They seemed to make some headway, although I do wonder how much they actually got accomplished or if it turned out to be more of a "visit."

We have also discussed what to do when she loses her hair. I'm all about having lots of options…a wig? A scarf? A hat? So, she's exploring options and giving it some thought. And I'm sure she will come up with what will be most comfortable for her. Of course, I put in my two cents-worth and said that if she does a wig, it has to be a good one. But hey, it will also save money – think of all the hair coloring Mom won't need to do for a while. Gotta find that silver lining wherever you can!

This past week was full of more doctors' appointments, and I know it's wearing thin for Mom. I think she's about had it with all the bloodwork, CT scans, scheduling her surgery for the port, etc. She met with Dr. Loftus, the vascular surgeon who will insert her port and that surgery (outpatient) is scheduled for Wednesday afternoon. That will be a walk in the park after everything else she's been through.

All in all, it was a pretty good week. Although I must say, she's spent so much time trying to write out all her Christmas/Holiday/New Year/Thank You cards (it's an all-in-one card this year). That's been so important to her and I'm hoping she is about done, so we can go out and do some fun things! So, if you haven't received a card, I'm sure it will be on its way shortly; she just finished them.

I think the biggest highlight for Mom last week was making the trek down to Concord (at my gentle urging) to see my niece Gabriella play basketball for Carondelet High School. It's her senior year and this was the first home game of their regular season, which is just getting underway. Yes, and Mom was all dolled up and sporting her red CHS basketball fleece pullover. I know it wasn't an easy day for her (she has good days and then some real challenging ones), but I'm sure that the joy she got in watching Gab play and having QT (quality time) with Dom and Janine at the game made it all worthwhile. Oh, and of course, Gab had a great game and they won! Even better. She can add that to the "memory bank."

Last Thursday was a very tough day. Mom had to do another CT scan and that one really did a number on her. She was so sick and we're guessing it was from the "potion" she had to drink along with the dye that they injected her with. Either way, I'm pretty sure she won't be doing a CT scan again for a very, very long time. If she has her way, that will have been her last one!

Then on Sunday afternoon, Mom suggested we take a little walk down by the Napa River. And what better way to celebrate our 49er victory than with a little "happy dance" down Main Street? (I'll get to that in a minute.) It was a beautiful afternoon (just a bit breezy) and the perfect day for a stroll and to get out of the house. I've wanted to see the 9/11 Memorial, so we made a little stop there. Very impressive and I highly recommend that everyone pay a visit to see this beautiful and very thoughtful memorial if you're ever in the area. Oh, and then we ventured over to check out the "cha cha" steps that are in downtown Napa. That was so fun! It is an art installation that has been donated by the artist if I understand correctly (it's embedded in the sidewalk).

So, there we were – doing the cha cha celebration dance on Main Street! Yes, another moment for the memory bank.

So, to close out, the new week is upon us with more doctors' appointments (to review the CT scan and lab work), a chemo class to attend (who knew you had to take a class?), and the minor surgery port placement. All this to be done before Mom starts chemo, which is scheduled for Tuesday, January 21. A busy week it will be, but she's doing great and getting stronger day by day!

CHAPTER 10

CHEMO CLASS

Saturday, January 25
Phase 2 Underway

Ok, I realize that I'm really slacking in my reporting and updates. Been over a week and I have no idea where the time has gone! But I do have updates...and all good ones! Right now, as I'm typing my mom and dad are at Gabriella's basketball game (I'm guessing all dolled up in her Carondelet basketball #11 blinged-out shirt) as Carondelet takes on another great team, St. Mary's of Berkeley. I am in Las Vegas right now getting ready to list my home for sale and while I'm not at home with Mom, I now know how to gauge how she is feeling. If there's a game of Gab's or Dom's and she's feeling ok, I know she'll be there. If anyone wants to see Mom, maybe you should get a copy of the Carondelet varsity basketball schedule!

And you can pretty much count on Mom being there, unless she's under the weather.

Let me back up now for a minute...to January 14. Mom and I attended her "chemo class" with two of the oncology nurses and I must say, once again, the level of service provided is incredible. Teresa and Jenny reviewed and discussed with Mom all the "do's and don't's" and "what if's" of what we can expect. Much is still unknown, as we'll just have to wait and see how Mom handles her special concoction of chemo drugs – Carboplatin and Taxol. More information to store in the memory bank.

Then, on January 15, Mom and I were at the Queen of the Valley Hospital for her outpatient surgery to have the port inserted. Yes, it was another day of adventure in the hospital...we discovered the newest technology with these heatable gowns (which allow you to control the flow of hot or cold air). So fun to pump some air through and adjust the temp setting as you need! Mom's team that day: Robin (her nurse), Dr. Loftus (the surgeon), and Dr. Yamanishi (the anesthesiologist with the cute and colorful scrub hat!). They were all so amazing!

So, there we were in Room 8 waiting for Mom to be summoned to the operating room when I happen to overhear a conversation down the hall. All I heard was "gunshot wound" followed by "yes, you'll be going into surgery soon." Well, of course, that piqued my curiosity and I decided to venture down the hall-way…and there they were – two law enforcement officers just two doors down, in Room 6. I couldn't get a very good look at the guy and decided that was probably for the best.

After Mom had her surgery (she did great), I was in the recovery room with her and then she tells me another story. Apparently, as she was coming out of her anesthesia, she heard someone say something about a 92-year-old man next to her. She asked the nurse if she heard that correctly and the nurse replied, "Yes, the man just had a circumcision." Now, I think I'll just leave that one alone – but it sure did give Mom and I some great conversation on the ride home! I then escaped for a little three-day "stay-cation" with 15 friends from Las Vegas who came to town.

So, a big shout out and thank you to all Mom's friends who brought her food. The refrigerator was loaded with such good food!

Then, on Sunday, January 19, Mom was up for a little drive…so we drove down to the El Cerrito Fire Department to visit Joe for his birthday. His captain, Brian Chesharek, spent all day cooking – smoking ribs! Mom thoroughly enjoyed the ribs, some mashed potatoes, salad, French bread, and, of course, a little birthday cake (but just a little piece!). It was such a special evening, and the only downside was that the 49ers lost to Seattle!

On Monday, January 20, Mom decided to have her hair done. Might be the last time she gets this done for a while, so we made the best of it. In fact, she had a totally unplanned little rendezvous with her friends Dar (getting her hair done too) and Jaime (who I ran into in front of Whole Foods). Then, later that evening, Mom felt well enough to attend a birthday party with her "tap sisters" for a little while. I'm so proud of her for trying to get out and enjoy herself! That's what makes this all worthwhile – having those special moments and memories that are just priceless.

The next day, Tuesday, January 21, was the start of "Phase 2" – chemo treatment. We're now underway and Mom did great! Her nurses Teresa and Jenny were there to help ease any anxiety and make sure she was comfortable. My only complaint was the heavy set man sitting two chairs down whose T-shirt was way too short, and he snored way too loud as he was passed out in his recliner. Note for future visits: bring Mom some headphones! Other than that, it was pretty quiet and peaceful and as good an experience as you could hope for. So, one treatment down and 17 to go. Yes, I'm counting.

The great news was that Mom felt good enough to take another little "trip." And before you knew it, there we were on our way down to Concord to see Gabriella play another basketball game vs. San Ramon Valley High School. Gab did amazing and scored 24 points! Joe and Janine were there, and it was such a great night (just wish Dom had been there). What a great little reward after her first day of chemo...another fabulous evening for Mom to put in her memory bank!

On Wednesday, January 22, I went to Las Vegas and am here until Monday morning. I'll catch up with Mom tomorrow and get the "update" on how she's doing and how her weekend was. But I thought that both my mom and my dad could use a little "gift" – a break from me for a few days. Ha! I'm hoping it was a great weekend for my mom and my dad...and now I'm looking forward to getting back to California and the new week that lies ahead.

Sunday, February 2
"Game Day Prep"

So, today was game day and Super Bowl Sunday...as I'm sure you can imagine, I was NOT cheering for the Seattle Seahawks (since they took our 49ers out of contention). In retrospect, I think an analogy and a comparison can be made between "game day" and Mom's cancer and treatment. You try to be as prepared as possible (offensively and defensively) because you're not sure what will be coming at you or when, and so you try to take it one play or day at a time. In a way, I guess every day is "game day" for Mom.

So, here's a little recap and update on how Mom's week went.

Last Monday, I flew back from Las Vegas (to put my house up for sale) and first on the agenda was to take Mom to see her oncologist. Good news to report! Her CA-125 marker is at 117. This is a far cry from her pre-surgery marker that was over 2,000 and her post-surgery marker at 169. So, 117 will be Mom's new baseline and the goal is to be under 35. Although Mom has lost a bit more weight than the doctor would like, he is very happy with all her levels and where she's at. Her appetite seems to be getting a little better and she's really trying her best to keep the weight up.

On Tuesday, Mom had chemo treatment #2. It was practically standing room only and quite busy when we got there at 11 am. Her nurses Teresa, Jenny, and Robbie were on their "A" game as usual. Mom did great and she seemed like a pro at handling all the IVs. She spent the time reading, working on her new laptop (a great time for her to practice!), and just relaxing. After her treatment, we went out to lunch for a little treat at Pacific Blues in Yountville...Mom loves her pork sliders!

Thursday and Friday, however, ended up being lousy days for Mom and I could tell she just wasn't feeling very well. I think we are all trying to learn, figure it out, and adapt as we go. I'm guessing the chemo is doing its job, so that makes for very long and exhausting days for her. So, on those days, we just adapt the game plan and ensure that she gets her rest. And as I constantly remind her, I also think it helps to have something to look forward to.

So, on Saturday afternoon, Mom rallied back and we hit the road, once again, to go see Gabriella play another exciting game of basketball. Carondelet played Deer Valley and Joe, Janine, and Dom were all there (which made it extra special). Of course, Gab had a great game and afterwards she said that maybe Mom and I bring her good luck because she always plays great when we are there. I would like to think that there's a little bit of truth there! But what I do know is that Mom had a great afternoon. And although tiring for her with the hour plus drive each way, I know that it was a very special day filled with memorable moments and far outweighed the not-so-great previous two days. I think it is moments like the one we shared yesterday at Gab's game that make this difficult journey just a little more bearable. Certainly another one for the memory bank... so, here's to a new week and all that it holds.

Monday, February 10
Pay It Forward
Last week was truly a whirlwind of appointments, meetings, and more appointments. And it all began with Mom's weekly Monday appointment for blood-work and a brief meeting with the oncology doc. Mom's white blood cell (WBC) count is now in the low range (normal is between five and 10 and she

is at 2.2) and she is at risk of infection. Apparently, this is a common occurrence when one goes through chemo. So, Mom will now require Neupogen shots the day after chemo. This shot should help to stimulate production of the WBCs – but to Mom, I know it means another dreaded trip to the doctor's office.

On Tuesday, February 4, it was Mom's standing appointment in the infusion room – yep, chemo day. I gave Mom some space to chill out and relax in her recliner and just be. By the time I came back, I could see the bond forming between Mom and one of her nurses. Jenni is young, has tons of energy, is confident, incredibly knowledgeable and caring, and willing to spend quality time with Mom answering all her questions and helping to guide her through the unknown.

Jenni's from Iowa, so perhaps it's that Midwestern link they share. Whatever it is, it's truly special and I can see the calm come over Mom when she knows Jenni is there to help. Mom had a good chemo day and that was the end of her first cycle! Yay! However, the drugs do seem to be taking a toll. Mom continues to be very fatigued, but I guess that means the Carbo and Taxol are working and doing what they are supposed to do.

As part of our Tuesday routine, Mom took a rest when she got home from chemo and then in true Dolly fashion, she rallied in the evening. She wasn't going to miss out on all the festivities. It was my dad's birthday (I'm not saying a number!) and we all decided to venture down to Concord and see Gabriella's basketball game. So, we left early and drove down to meet Joe, Janine, and Dom for a great sushi dinner! (To our surprise, Dom skipped out on his baseball conditioning session – he will never pass up a sushi meal!) From there, we drove over to CHS to see Gab play another great game of basketball. She had a stunning 17 points and too many steals and assists for me to count. Let's just say her stats were great! I know it was a special birthday evening for my dad and was just such a fun and festive evening with the family all together. Yes, another one for the memory bank.

Last Wednesday was another special day for Mom – a reunion of sorts. Finally, the "Fab 5" get together (although it was just four because Carol was in Arizona for the birth of her granddaughter). They are long overdue, and it's been since my grandmother's funeral on November 12 that they were together. So, there at Trancas Steakhouse, a little local favorite spot, were the ladies – Sheilah, Donna, Marianne, and Mom all with their big bags filled with wrapped presents in tow – yes, they were ready to finally celebrate Christmas together!

There was nonstop chatter and laughter all mixed in. They definitely had much catching up to do! And I was so proud of Mom. She was all dolled up with her hair and makeup done and she looked great! It was truly a sight to see them all together again. When I came back over two hours later to pick up Mom, it was such a precious moment to see them reminiscing about their crazy escapades together over the years, many of which revolved around their theater days together – getting leotards switched by accident (imagine one is quite tall, the other very small), wearing a costume backwards (and possibly revealing a little more than anticipated), having your fringe skirt fall down...and the stories go on and on. After lunch, I took Mom to get her Neupogen shot and that rounded out another very busy but good day.

Rounding out the week last Thursday, was a "drive" with Aunt Beth and Mom to Pleasanton to visit Gary at his Gary Patrick hair salon. Through an acquaintance, I have befriended a woman here in Napa (in her early 50s) who, two years ago, went through ovarian cancer and all that goes with it – surgery, chemo, etc. Her name is Shawna, and she is truly special – incredibly thoughtful, caring, and willing to help someone she doesn't even know. She told me that she wanted to pay it forward (as someone had done for her when she was battling ovarian cancer), so she arranged for my mom to get an appointment the next day to meet Gary at his salon. All we had to do was show up. And that is how it's done!

So, we drove down to this salon that was hustling and bustling with energy. Come to find out that Gary himself is a cancer survivor and he knows all about hair loss and how it affects a person. He also knows how to treat and handle your hair as it's going through chemo treatment and beyond. He doesn't advertise this at all, but he helps people who are dealing with hair loss due to cancer treatments, alopecia, etc. He was able to explain to Mom what was happening to her hair as a result of the chemo (and by now it's shedding like crazy) as well as describe how she could take control of the situation (and not wait for it to get so bad that she's miserable). I called this "Operation Hair Overhaul," as we could see the progression of hair loss – it was getting worse by the day.

Long story short, Gary recommended that Mom shave her head sooner rather than later (within the next day or two) and she could come back with a wig for him to work with and he would get her all taken care of. And that is exactly what he did. He fit us in the next afternoon (Mom got a wig) and made the transition as painless as possible. Afterward, she celebrated with a glass of champagne! By the way, I actually think she has a great head. No weird shape at all! And it makes her eyes stand out. Not sure you'll ever see her like that, so you'll just have to take my word for it.

So, Mom now has options to play with...hair, no hair, hats, turbans, whatever. But the important take away here is that none of this would have happened if a woman that I barely know hadn't paid it forward to someone she's never met. How great is that? I know that Shawna and Mom will meet someday soon, and they will bond in ways that none of us can relate to (unless you've been through it). But one thing I promise to do is pay it forward in the same way that Shawna paid it forward to us. It is the least I can do.

Monday, February 17
It's All in the Numbers

Just a quick recap from the past week on Mom's progress and her activities. As usual, it was a crazy, busy week and this woman has me chauffeuring all over town!

The week got off to a great start on Tuesday morning when Mom went in for her chemo treatment. My brother Joe had offered to come up and take Mom to her chemo. He would take my chair for the morning ritual. So, he ventures off to Napa to spend some quality time together and he's come prepared – iPad and noise-canceling headphones in tow! Now, I wasn't there for this little incident...so I'm just recounting it as it was told to me.

Apparently, the doc came into the infusion room and handed Mom a piece of paper. He didn't say a word (he didn't have to) and just walked away with a little smirk on his face. Well, you see, that piece of paper said it all. Mom's CA-125 marker is now at 10! When I saw it, I asked the same question Mom did, "Are you sure this is right?" The doc knew he wouldn't have to say a word to Mom and that she would get it. In essence, the drugs are working...her marker's gone from 169 to 117 to 10.

Although her white blood cell counts are still really low, they are working on that with the Neupogen shots. And she's been taking precautions to prevent catching any little bug or infection. So, I'd say this was just a little proof to Mom that the chemo is working. I think the doc sensed a bit of concern and figured he would put her skepticism to rest. If not, I'm sure she'll inquire further when she sees the doc tomorrow!

Needless to say, Joe and Mom had a great morning together and then I arrived for the "changing of the guard."

After a "double dose" of chemo – this was Day 1 of Cycle 2, and she got both chemo drugs – Mom came home to rest, as she seemed really tired. I call it the "combo day" and this one seems to really hit her hard. But as Dolly does best, she rallied and we made it a family affair as my mom, my dad, and I drove down to Danville to catch the big match-up basketball game between Monte Vista and Carondelet.

Gabriella had a rough night, and it wasn't

one of her better games (I'll just leave it at that). Nevertheless, Mom had a great time at the game and the first half was quite exciting and intense (I could have used one of her Ativan pills to calm my nerves just from watching). But in true CHS fashion, they won by 20+ points. It really was a great family evening with Joe, Janine, and my mom and dad. The only missing link was Dom (he wasn't up for going to the game and I'm sure the teenager in him likes his freedom at home).

On Wednesday, Mom and I were busy doing a little wig shopping. We discovered the cutest little baseball hats and they'll be great to give her a few more options. Oh, she is all set for baseball season with Dom now! We're ready to play ball!

Thursday through Sunday were pretty tough for Mom. Just no energy at all and very taxing for her. But Thursday was a very special day as it was my mom and my dad's 49th wedding anniversary. Mom got all dolled up and looked fabulous for her celebratory dinner at Bistro Jeanty. Yes, I must admit that I crashed that party, too! I was going to give them a quiet dinner for two by the fireplace...but then they invited me. And well, I just couldn't resist! And yes, it was a magical and very special evening for my mom and dad together!

Today, I think Mom was going a bit stir crazy from being cooped up in the house the past few days and needed a little "excursion." So, as I write this, my mom and my dad are en route over to my Aunt Beth and Uncle Keith's house for a visit and to enjoy a nice evening out of the house.

Monday, February 24
Acts of Kindness

This morning, it's a beautiful blue-sky day in Las Vegas...yes, I said Las Vegas. I'm back in Nevada for the "pack and move" job. One of the positive aspects of moving is that you get to "clear the clutter" and feel like you're starting anew.

Anyway, here's a little rewind to last week...which was chemo week #5. As usual, Mom was greeted by her nurses – Mayra, Jenni, and Theresa. She's getting the royal treatment and it was a day all about "resting," as she's quite fatigued these days. So, she rested and reclined in her big chair...most memorable for me that day was looking up to check on Mom and there she was..."air" toe-tapping to the music – some musical or Broadway tune! Totally cracked me up.

After her treatment, we drove straight down to Concord. Yes, it was Tuesday – Gabriella's basketball night. Her game was in the DLS gym and Gab had a much better game, which I think was helped by Mom's cheering her on. A nice surprise was to see Ray and Betty Marchetti there – dear friends of the family.

Perhaps you are all starting to figure out that if you want to see Mom, catch her at one of Gab's or Dom's sporting events!

On Wednesday, Mom had a doctor's appointment with her new primary doctor, Dr. Jewell. Ok, he's another adorable, young, with-it, and very sharp doctor. Low and behold, another surprise! Who do we run into? Her dear friend (and now mine) Terri Gardella, a nurse at Queen of the Valley Hospital. Only in Napa could you sit in the doctor's office for almost an hour to catch up and get all the updates. Terri, you know how much we love you and you have done so much to help my mom with all her doctors.

Thursday and Friday were pretty much "rest" days, as Mom was conserving her energy to gear up for the big basketball game on Friday night. It was Gabriella's last home game as a Carondelet Cougar and we were all going to be there for "Senior Night" (my mom, my dad, Joe, Janine, and Dom). What an amazing tribute made to the three senior girls on the team. And after the game they had a dinner, presentation, and even a little entertainment for the families and the team. So, I'm sure Friday wiped her out...but she hung in there and I think really enjoyed the evening of having the family all together. The weekend I'm sure was a restful one for both my mom and my dad, as the house was soon quiet without me coming and going. I'm checking in on her daily and will get the updates for the week.

Gab is now in post-season playoff games for the Northern California Section, so I'm sure Mom will try and get to those games this week with my dad.

In closing, today my message is one of gratitude and celebration for the acts of kindness bestowed upon me. One of my very best friends, Sylvie, has flown to Las Vegas from Montreal to help me move. She's classically French - Canadian in every sense of the word and just an amazing woman. Why on earth would someone want to come thousands of miles to help me pack up? It's really not a fun job. I think the major advantage and selling point I had going for me is that it enabled her to escape the ridiculous cold of northern Canada! She's recently been working at a job in the province of Labrador in -45-degree weather (yes, that was a negative number).

But I can't say "merci" enough to my amazing and incredibly special friend...oh yes, everyone should have a French-Canadian friend on board when they move – the dining is fabulous! Homemade oat bran muffins in the morning...gourmet meals in the evening with a glass of red wine, etc. It sure makes moving a little more bearable! With that, I'm off to go pack a few more boxes today...wishing you all a wonderful week ahead and may you, too, see little acts of kindness flourish around you. Au revoir!

Sunday, March 9
A Treadmill of Fun

So, I'm back from Las Vegas and, of course, the treadmill continues. But I must confess, it's been a "treadmill of fun" this past week! Mom is doing well and hanging in there. She's seven for 18 with chemo treatments and just shy of the halfway mark. Fatigue continues to be the biggest challenge and Mom is trying to manage this balancing act. But I must confess, we do have the tendency to sometimes overdo it! This past week was jam-packed with appointments and activities.

On Wednesday, Mom decided she wanted to hit the church for Ash Wednesday and what a wonderful morning! We hadn't been to church since my grandmother's funeral, so it was a bittersweet visit. But Mom had a lovely reunion after with her friends at church – Sharon, Bobbi, Melinda, and Norma. Then after, Mom was up for some breakfast and was craving her omelet – I've got her now yearning for protein! So, we ventured over to Pacific Blues and being the small town that it is, we ran into Betty Jake. Another little reunion and homecoming for Mom! This is why I love to get her out and about, so that she can be surrounded by all her wonderful friends. And yes, Betty, I did break my "rule" and let Mom have a little ketchup with her eggs.

On Thursday, Mom had a follow-up with her surgeon Dr. Lerner. He said Mom is doing well considering everything that she's been through and he's continuing to keep an eye on her. At one point, though, I noticed Mom got that little glimmer in her eye and then I knew – here it comes – the inquisition! She dove right in and diverted the conversation away from her and back to him, asking him all about the upcoming wedding plans for September. I swear she is going to crash his wedding! And I know she'll expect me to be the accomplice "driver." We are teetering on the edge of reason here and I'm not sure I can contain this one.

On Friday evening, Mom got all dolled up and we went to see the production of "Annie Get Your Gun" with 13 of her nearest and dearest Napa tappers (one of their own, Dar, was performing in the show and she did great). Everyone was so excited for this little "reunion," and it was such a fabulous evening. Yes, there we all were spread out in Row F. And as exhausted as she was, Mom had put together cards and flowers for all the performers that she knew. What a great show with such a talented group. Definitely worth checking out if you're in the Napa area!

After the show, it was a major gab fest and catch-up chat session for Mom and all her friends. It practically took an act of Congress to get her out of there. It was way past our bedtime when we got home and I'm pretty sure she had a good night's sleep from all the activity that day. Needless to say, I gave Mom strict instructions to get lots of rest on Saturday because she had another big evening ahead. Gabriella was playing in the North Coast championship basketball game at St. Mary's College, and I knew there was no way that Mom was going to miss out on this one.

I was down in Walnut Creek for the day to catch Dom's double-header baseball game, so Aunt Beth and Uncle Keith came by to pick up my mom and my dad and they all went out for a pre-game dinner – and then we all met at the gym for the big game. It was a packed gym, and the energy was running high.

Of course, Joe, Janine, Dom, and I were all there along with some of Janine's family. And it was so great to see Maynard and Sharon Clark join in to catch the action. As they have also figured out, it's a great way to see my mom and my dad, too! Even Robin Krill and her daughter Lindsay came all the way down from Napa to check out the game (Lindsay plays basketball for Justin-Siena High School). The championship game was against Clayton Valley High School and ended up being a bit of a blowout. CHS was "en fuego" and just couldn't be stopped. They scored 100 points and are the new North Coast Champions! We are looking forward to hopefully making it all the way to the California state championships! The next game is scheduled for this Friday with CHS vs. Sacred Heart of San Francisco (game being played at De La Salle). So today – Sunday – was declared Mom's "day of rest and recovery," so she can be ready for another busy and active memory-making week!

Wednesday, March 19
Single Digits and a Social Calendar

The life of Dolly only continues to get busier and crazier as the weeks go by. I'm figuring that Mom is getting into her "chemo groove" and has figured out her "good" vs. "bad" days. My mission was to get mom out and about and truly living her life (as we have all known her to do). Well, MISSION ACCOMPLISHED. I'm exhausted! Over the past few weeks, it's been a whirlwind of non-stop activities.

On March 11, Mom wanted to see her tennis team play their last home match vs. Meadowood. She went so far as to get her chemo appointment pushed back, so she could cheer on the Napa "royal blues" in action! Mom was dolled up in her team color sweats and was greeted by lots of hugs, laughter, and love. I even got an "I love you" shout out from someone on her team who was in the middle of match play! And there I was on the sidelines chatting with two of her teammates, Helen and Diana, when the conversation came up about her doctors. Let's just say Dr. Dugan has his own little fan club of admirers!

From there, we high-tailed it over to the chemo center and checked in. As usual, Jenni had Mom all set up with her "corner lounge chair" (Mom's favorite) and without fail, delivered wonderful care and put any of Mom's worries to rest. Well, the not-so-good news is that we found out Jenni's moving to

Georgetown Hospital in Washington, DC for a more permanent position in their oncology dept. Mom and I are already scheming on how we can derail her departure until Mom's done with chemo. Jenni says her last day is April 11, so that doesn't leave us with much time for a game plan to "re-route" her back to Napa.

Oh, and last Thursday, Mom did a little "escape" on her own. Well, not really. I must confess that I went out of town for a long weekend (took Dom and Joe to Spring Training Baseball in Arizona for Dom's Christmas present – Christmas in March!). And of course, as soon as I depart, Mom's got her agenda going and calendar filling up! That day she drove and went to see her tennis team in action again. I can only imagine how much fun they all had getting together. I'll be shocked if they actually got much tennis playing in!

Other than that, it was a relaxing weekend for Mom to just recuperate and get ready for the busy week ahead. Although she and my dad did go over to Aunt Beth and Uncle Keith's house for a little pre- St. Paddy's Day dinner. I don't even want to know the sugar content of that dinner...all I know is that it ended with an "Irish coffee or two." My Aunt Beth can be a very bad influence (but in a good way, of course!).

Even though it's only Wednesday, this week has been nuts! On Tuesday, Mom had chemo and this was a milestone accomplishment. She is halfway through her treatments, and we are now in the single digits – nine weeks to go! It was a challenging day and Mom found out that her red blood cell count is really low and that she would need a blood transfusion. So, after chemo, we had to go over to the hospital for her blood test to be done – a cross and type match – so that she could have her transfusion. We literally left at 10am and didn't get home until 3pm, where we were greeted by my dad, Aunt Beth, and Uncle Keith. We immediately had to refresh and change into our "basketball uniforms," get in the car, and get on the road to get down to Concord for an early sushi dinner before watching Gabriella play in the CIF state playoffs. And well, tonight was going to be what many considered THE biggest game of the year – Carondelet vs. Miramonte and the game was at De La Salle.

Somehow, Joe arranged to get sponsors and "6th Man" t-shirts made for everyone in attendance as well as having energy-pumping music flowing through the gym. It was absolute high energy and noise levels through the roof! It was a game for the record books! It was absolutely packed and wall-to-wall people. The only downside was that the Cougars fell short last night: 92-87. The silver lining was that Gab had a great game and played her heart out. 15 points, rebounds, steals, and some incredible assists made her a top contributor to her team (and I'm not just saying that because she's my niece!).

News flash: She also made the EBAL All-Star team. Needless to say, there were lots of friends and family there to join in the festivities and I know that Mom enjoyed it immensely. We didn't get home until almost 10:30pm and I knew we had another busy day that would commence in just a few hours.

Today, Mom had to be at the hospital for a 9am appointment for her blood transfusion. Two units and over four hours later, Mom then had to jaunt off to meet "The Fab Five" for their "Christmas lunch get together." Because Carol was MIA last time, they had another "date" scheduled for this afternoon at Bistro Don Giovanni in Napa. Then, Mom had to go and get her Neupogen shot. She finally rolled in the door after 5 pm this evening and I can say that she's now got her head on the pillow and hopefully in a dream state!

So, I'm sure you get the picture now – her calendar just keeps filling up and it's one great activity after another! I'm exhausted just writing all this, but with a definite smile on my face. I love seeing Mom push the limits to get the most out of every day. I know that sometimes it's a bit too much for her and she overdoes it, but at the end of the day I know she's loving all the quality time spent with family and friends. Next up, Dom and his baseball season! The season is underway and I'm hoping she'll be up for a game this weekend in Walnut Creek.

So, I'm happy to report that we're on the downhill

slope and Mom has only nine more treatments to go! Of course, I'm sure she's still got that calendar filling up and I wouldn't want it any other way.

Sunday, March 30
Another Whirlwind Week

So, a week has passed by and, yet again, Mom has outdone herself. This past Tuesday marked treatment #10 and a challenging "double dose" chemo week (these seem to be the hardest). I know she felt pretty lousy, but, somehow, she picked herself up by the bootstraps and pushed onward. I swear she just doesn't want to miss out on anything. So, of course, there are lots of activities and events to update you on!

It all began on Friday, March 21, when I woke up in the morning, came into the kitchen, and realized that Mom had "escaped" yet again. She was nowhere to be found, her car was missing, and there was no note. (I thought she'd at least leave me a note. Talk about a role reversal...perhaps it's payback for all the times I kept her worrying because I was out late. Around 9 am, she comes waltzing in with a little skip in her step – she had just been to church.

On Saturday, I went down to check out Dom's double header baseball game and gave Mom a day to rest and hang out with my dad. Later that night my mom and my dad had "date night" (no, I did not crash that party) and they drove up to Twin Pines for a little dinner and some slot action! A little entertainment and so nice to get out of the house for an evening.

The next afternoon, Aunt Beth, Uncle Keith, and Uncle Steve came over for a little BBQ in the afternoon. It was such a gorgeous day, and we just couldn't pass up having my dad do a little grilled chicken on the barbie...and, of course, Mom was in the kitchen with me doing way more than she should. We had some pasta and grilled veggies to round out the meal and even some brownies for dessert (yes, they were sugar free!).

The next day was an absolutely much-needed day of rest for Mom. I think perhaps she may have overdone it, but I'm guessing she wouldn't have changed a thing.

So, then rolls around Tuesday...March 25 and chemo day. I swear I'm calling it "Chatty Cathy Tuesday" – those steroids do a little number on her and get her all revved up! At dinner, between my mom and my dad, I couldn't get a word in edgewise. So, I just sat back and enjoyed the show. I tell you, Mom talked so much that she wore herself out! Unfortunately, she ends up roaming through the house at the wee hours of the morning and that is when you may get some interesting emails from her.

Part of our "family dinnertime conversation" includes making plans for the week's activities – Dom's baseball game on Wednesday (weather permitting) and pay a visit to Terri and Lacey, her new eight-week-old Golden Retriever puppy in the afternoon. If the baseball game is canceled, then the back up plan is to go to Sonoma and meet my Aunt Beth and cousin Terri for dinner – and then if all still goes well, go see Sheilah who's performing in the play "Social Security." Yes, the schedule is packed!

On Wednesday, Mom was sluggish and feeling pretty lousy. But, somehow, I coerce her into getting out of the house – or maybe she was just having some "cabin fever." But how could you not have a great day that starts with visiting an adorable puppy? So, off and running we went...grabbed Lacey some treats and toys and we paid "the girls" a visit. So fun to hang out with Terri Gardella and just watch Lacey, a precious little Golden Retriever, in action.

From there, we headed over to Sonoma (Dom's baseball game was canceled) and met Aunt Beth and Terri for dinner at Ledsen Hotel. We sat by the fireplace on a cold and chilly evening and enjoyed a fabulous evening of food, wine, and conversation. What an absolutely great time we had! Of course, we didn't stop there. Oh no, Aunt Beth and Terri have us strolling down the street, turning down an alley, and before you know it, we are in Murphy's Irish Pub. It was Wednesday Night Trivia! Gary (Terri's boyfriend) met us there and, before you know it, there's Mom and Aunt Beth sipping on their Baileys

Irish Cream and partaking in trivia. We didn't win, but we didn't come in last either. We'll look forward to doing this again, but next time we'll make sure to study up on our state capitols, Saturn's moons, and the United Nations! We got home late that night and it's great to see Mom sleeping in a little bit more each morning.

On Thursday, Mom treated herself to her first mani and pedi and I knew it'd be a relaxing and calming day for her. She's all polished up and I'm sure you're wondering where she's off to next. Well, later that evening, she had the "Tappers Birthday Dinner Soirée." See, there are about 15 of them in this group and they all get together to celebrate their birthdays. This month it was Darleen Bevin, Connie Courtright, Jamie Hunt, and Andrea Biocca. Happy birthday, ladies!!!

Mom strolled in after 9:30pm and, of course, I'm sure her head hit that pillow pretty hard! Friday and Saturday were tough days, so Mom was layin' low and taking it easy. She had to rest up for the next event on her calendar...seeing Sheilah Morrison perform in "Social Security."

This afternoon, Aunt Beth, Mom, and I ventured out to Antioch at the El Campanil Theatre and caught the closing show. All I can tell you is that Sheilah was absolutely hilarious! Her first scene onstage – she makes her entrance, doesn't say a word, and I'm absolutely cracking up (you have to see her in action). I'm laughing so hard, I have tears in my eyes. If you know the story, she plays an elderly, aging Jewish mother who's living with her daughter and son-in-law for a while. Let's just say that in my eyes, Sheilah stole the show! And I might add, she does a great little "strip scene" number onstage that was just classic!

FYI, Sheilah will be in The Cemetery Club in November and I can promise you that we'll be there to see her in that, too. The woman is talented – you don't get 11 Shellie Award nominations for nothing. So, be on the lookout for her performing in a neighborhood near you. She's not to be missed!

After the show, Aunt Beth, Mom, and I went to dinner at my new favorite Yountville spot – R+D Kitchen. They never disappoint and it's a little hot spot bustling with high energy! The perfect end to a wonderful, exhausting, and fun-filled week. Mom will most certainly be getting her rest tomorrow as she prepares for yet another busy week ahead.

CHAPTER 11

KEEPING SECRETS

Saturday, April 19
Light at the End of the Tunnel

Ok, so I've heard through the grapevine that a few of you out there are wondering how Mom is doing. I really haven't forgotten you! I was MIA for a week and then came back to being crazy busy (as usual). I decided to "escape" for a little rest and relaxation (I was starting to get a little snappy with my parents and knew that it was time to exit stage right). So, I took a little getaway and was gone from March 30-April 7 in Riviera Maya, Mexico.

It was great fun, but not as relaxing as antici-pated. My girlfriend Carla joined me and we found ourselves on day trips of snorkeling with the sea turtles, sightseeing at Tulum, spending a day in the jungle rappelling down into these cenotes (world's largest underwater river system), zip lining, snorkeling in the cenotes, spending a day sailing on a catamaran over to Isla Mujeres, snorkeling in the national park (fabulous!), etc. So much for chilling out on the beach reading a book! I didn't have phone access, but was able to touch base with Mom via email. I made it clear to her that no matter where I was in the world, I was expecting to be kept in the loop and updated on her progress. Well, she claimed that all was well and that it was a pretty "boring" week.

She lied to me! It wasn't until I returned that I found out she'd been in ER that Friday night with a required "sleepover." All of you accomplices out there that kept this from me – I know who you are! Although I certainly understand why you did it. When I got back and found out from Pop what had happened, Mom couldn't see my "blood boiling over" because I have a good tan going right now. But I know that she knows how I feel about it all. Enough said.

Even Mom's nurses were nervously asking her "Have you told Lizann yet?"

So, when I accompanied Mom to chemo treatment #12 (on April 8), the nurses were all treading very lightly and giving me a little look as if to say, "Do you know?" Yeah, well, the cat was out of the bag, and I finally got the scoop.

Luckily, that Friday (April 4) my dad was taking her to get her "f***ing Neupogen shot" (as I refer to it now), when the nurses noticed she was quite pale, didn't feel well, and lo and behold once they took her vitals, they knew something was wrong. It's the same issue she had in ICU right after her surgery – her heart goes into A-fib (atrial fibrillation).

Long story short, they got her over to the ER right away and, luckily for her, her heart flipped back over (so, she didn't need the shock treatment). Although right about now, I think she needs a good shock for keeping this all from me! My dad was a trooper and was with her throughout the entire ordeal. What continues to impress me the most was the care that she received from her doctors – both oncology doctors (Dr. Dugan and Dr. Ari) came by the hospital to check on her, the cardio doc made an appearance, and even her primary care physician Dr. Jewell came by to check on her (love that guy!). So, if nothing else, I know without a doubt that she is in great hands, and lots of them!

Suffice to say, I was determined to get Mom out and about during the week and to make sure that she had some fun activities and events to look forward to.

It's never a dull moment with my niece and nephew and they provide us with so many of our excursions! That Wednesday (April 9), Mom and I drove out to Concord to catch Dom's baseball game with Joe and Janine in attendance, too. He did great, we all had a blast, and then we all went out to dinner (even Gab came to meet us). It was a night full of high energy and lots of laughs (especially seeing Gab right after her spray tan in prep for her Senior Ball – let's just say her teeth were glowing in the dark). What better way to spend a lovely evening than with family? The only one missing was my dad, which was a bummer. But I don't hold it against him, as Wednesdays are a lot of "car time" for him going down to work in Emeryville and back. But I'm holding out that one of these days I'll get him down there with us for a weeknight game!

On Friday, Mom and I had to go see the nurses – not because she needed another f***ing Neupogen shot, but because she had to say goodbye to Jeni... the amazing nurse that Mom has formed a very special bond with. I tried to talk her out of leaving, but her family easily beat me on this one. She's decided to move back to Des Moines, Iowa to be closer to her family. She's tired of all the traveling and ready to settle down a bit.

So, Mom and I made a surprise visit and left her with a parting gift – the exact same blanket that Mom uses when she's in the infusion room. Jeni would always come over and "pet the oh-so-soft leopard print blanket." We found the absolute perfect gift for Jeni. My hope is that every time she sees it or uses it (which she will in those Iowa winters!), she'll think of Mom and the special bond they share, and I know it'll continue across the miles. She was so sweet and even gave Mom her cell phone number (which she does not give out easily). Mom was always full of questions and Jeni said that if Mom ever had questions, she could always email or call. I can honestly say, I miss her already!

The following day, Saturday, April 12, was another adventure...my Aunt Beth accompanied us down to Alamo to see Gab, her friends, and all their dates – all dolled up for the CHS/DLS Senior Ball. All I can tell you is that I want a "do over" on the Senior Ball. These kids go all out! Boy, have times changed. The dresses are gorgeous, and the girls are totally dolled up (hair, makeup, eyelashes, nails, spray tan). I thought I was going to the Miss California Pageant! I know Mom loved every minute of it (as did we all). The first stop was to see Gab with her best friends – Gianna, Molly, and Kylie all together with their dates (we met at Molly's house). From there, we drove over to Oakhurst Country Club in Clayton...where more kids gathered "with their clans" to take photos together. It was a beautiful setting overlooking the golf course and overflowing with kids and parents. Then we saw two luxury buses pull up that would take these two groups to San Francisco for their big event at the Westin St. Francis. From there, Aunt Beth, Mom, and I drove back to Napa and had a great little dinner recapping the day's festivities at Bistro Don Giovanni.

On Sunday, I ventured down to Walnut Creek to see Dom play in a double-header baseball game and gave my parents a "day of rest" without me. What did they do? They took a little drive up to Calistoga and then had dinner out at Tra Vigne.

On Monday, April 14, we drove down to St. Mary's College in Moraga to show our support for Janine and her family. We were attending the funeral service of her father Chuck Bellia, who was finally at peace after a long struggle with illness. What a beautiful service and reception they organized, and it was nice to have all our family together in a supportive manner during this difficult time. We got home that evening, and I can honestly say that we tuckered Mom out with a week of activities!

This past Tuesday, April 15, marked Mom's chemo treatment #13. It was a tough one – the double dose day – so, it's been a difficult week for her and one in which her time has been spent doing a few errands… but mostly just relaxing.

Aunt Beth did come over on Wednesday and she and Mom were quite busy organizing and clearing the clutter. But Mom is doing great and her CA-125 marker is down to 7.5 (which is fabulous!), so that is all positive news. And of course, it's Easter Sunday tomorrow and there is Mom busy trying to get little gifts wrapped.

In closing, the other day I looked at Mom, smiled, and said, "You know, you only have five more treatments to go. I can see the light at the end of the tunnel."

She gave me her big smile and I know that she can see the light, too. Here's wishing you all a very special and Happy Easter spent with your beloved family and friends!

Sunday, May 11
A Very Special Mother's Day
It's Sunday afternoon, May 11, and the troops have departed and gone their separate ways...I find myself sitting outside alone on the patio and relaxing overlooking the vineyards with a nice, cool breeze blowing through. Today, as usual, it's been quite a busy day! It is Mother's Day after all, and we've had a plethora of activities keeping us busy...more to share on that a bit later. My apologies for not keeping you all updated on Mom's progress over these past few weeks. You'll see how busy we've been from all that I'm about to share. So, grab a seat and settle in for a good little update.

Three weeks ago, exactly, it was Easter Sunday and I must confess it wasn't our "normal" celebration. We didn't make it to Mass, as Mom was just too exhausted. The last couple of weeks are definitely taking its toll and it's the culmination of 15+ weeks of chemo all adding up. I tried to make it a very special Easter for Mom, even though I knew she felt like crap. So, I whipped up some blueberry pancakes with my favorite syrup – Walden Farms (and it has no sugar, calories, etc). It's the best! Then, Connie stopped by to say "hi" and deliver her Easter bunny chocolates (I made an exception on this one day for Mom to have some chocolate. I know Connie is aware of my "sugar rules" – but when she just smiles and gives me that cute little laugh, I can't help but give in). She even bribed me with a chocolate Easter bunny!

That afternoon, we trekked down to Lafayette for a lovely Easter brunch at my cousin's house. It was brimming with kids, high energy, great food, and laughter! It was a wonderful day well spent with family and when Mom got home she was just exhausted.

The next day, Mom and I decided to hit the road, get out of the house, and go to the movies. She got her popcorn (butter and all) and cozied into the theater to see "Heaven Is for Real." Wow, what a touching true story that just kept us enraptured. At the end of the movie Mom told me that when she was in the hospital for her surgery, she didn't go to heaven. But then she immediately came back with,

"But I didn't go to hell either."

Then on Tuesday, it was chemo treatment day (#14) – and a great day to hear from Theresa, her nurse, that Mom's white blood cell count was great – and that she wouldn't need any Neupogen shots that week. Woo hoo! We get our celebrations in lots of small, tiny victories. And we were takin' this one! That meant Mom didn't have to go back to the doc's office for the rest of the week.

On Wednesday, April 23, Aunt Beth came over for a visit. Of course, I should have known that she would bring over some not-so-healthy pumpkin bread for Mom...but I let it slide again for the day. I know how much Mom loves having that with her coffee in the morning.

Together, Mom with her posse in tow, we ventured over to the tennis courts to watch and support Mom's tennis team. They were playing for the Napa/Sonoma/Marin Division B2 3.5 Championships! What a sight to see at 9:30am – matches on all the courts going on, hugs and kisses abound at the sight of Mom (dressed in her team colors, eccentric tennis earrings, and who knows what other good luck charms she was donning). Today, she was their #1 cheerleader! So, with her posse in tow, we head down to court #1 to check in on the action. All I can say is that one of the singles opponents (I'll call her the eccentric lady in purple) was causing quite a commotion with her antics. Apparently, she was distraught by all the "noise" and chatter – didn't we know we were supposed to whisper? Then, the high school kids came wheeling some grocery cart by the courts (I have no idea what they were up to) and the lady went off. Let's just say it was less than desirable to be her opponent! I think it was just as much of a mental as it was a physical match up. And I have to admit that I found myself "sideline coaching" in Aunt Beth's ear.

I was all engrossed and saying, "She should aim for the corners, hit one short and then long, make her run because the lady in purple can't run at all, hit to her backhand (I thought it was her weak side)."

I was absolutely possessed with this match. Finally, Mom said we had to go down to the other end and catch some of the doubles matches. Suffice to say, that singles match lasted over four hours! And good news – Patricia of the Napa team prevailed as the winner of that match.

Down at the other end of the courts, we were cheering on Kathy (Mom's former tennis partner) and all the gals playing. And then it was a roaring applause and cheers for Nancy Coursen and her partner. Not only did they win their match, but they also cinched the championship win for the team! Our emotions were running high, and I think it tuckered Mom out.

Then, we got home only to find out that Joe was there digging a grave under the big, wild walnut tree. Cinca (their wonderful yellow lab) had passed away that morning. Although it was heartbreaking to see another of our dogs join those who passed before her – Ty, Cozy, and Cody, she really had a very full life of 13 years. She was such a special dog...needless to say, I like to think that they are all together and running around in dog heaven!

Don't ask me how Mom had the energy, but she and Aunt Beth decided to escape for a little "slot therapy" as I like to say. The results were apparently less than desirable (hint: they lost and came home with pockets a little lighter), although I know that the journey was well worth it. Two sisters hanging out together and just having some good ol' fun! I'm guessing Mom slept pretty well that night from all the day's activities.

After a few days of down time, Joe and clan came up for a visit on Sunday, April 27. It always cheers us up when they come up for a visit. We get to catch up with the kids and find out the latest and greatest of what's happening in their lives.

On Monday, Mom had a doctor's appointment and then I decided we should go for a little drive up to the valley. It was such a nice afternoon and I carted Mom up to St. Helena to the Napa Valley Roasting Company for their famous cinnamon latte. We were able to just sit out on the patio and enjoy our drinks before making our way back home to crank up the BBQ for our first BBQ of the season!

On Tuesday, April 29, Mom had chemo treatment #15 followed by lunch at the Yountville Golf Course. What a gorgeous setting and fabulous view. It is a little gem of a local spot!

The next day, I ran errands and let Mom rest – as she had to save her energy for the next day.

On Thursday, she spent the day with the Queen – at the hospital that is (Queen of the Valley)! It was time for another blood transfusion, and it was an all-day affair. Luckily, Mom knew the drill and what to expect – so she went prepared with reading material, cards to write out, etc. Terri Gardella, a nurse at the hospital and a dear friend, stopped by to see Mom and I know that really perked her up! After all that, then Mom had to get her Neupogen shot. What a pain that little shot is! That weekend, Mom did a whole lot of relaxing and sleeping.

On Monday, May 5, my parents went to see Dr. Dugan for an update. What great news he delivered... Mom's treatment is going exactly as planned. Her CA-125 marker is down to 7.5, and she is almost done!

They actually had the "Ok, what's next after chemo?" conversation and the best news of all is that Mom can start living her life again. Silently,

I think she's scheming and will probably have all sorts of things planned that she wants to do, which is how it should be. I was bummed I wasn't there with them to hear that news, but I was otherwise engaged in my fifth interview with a company (trying to secure myself an elusive job in the Napa Valley).

On Tuesday, May 16, Mom had chemo treatment #16 and it was "double dose" and a very long day. This was her last "double dose" chemo! You see, she has 18 treatments planned and now only two to go. This double dose is a tough one and just takes a lot out of her. I swear it is that nasty carboplatin drug that wreaks all the havoc. And the steroids keep her up all night! But Mom, she rallied the next day and on Wednesday afternoon, we drove down to Walnut Creek to check out Dom's baseball game, followed by dinner with Janine and Dom. And Dom's choice for dinner – sushi! So fun to catch up with them and the conversation ranged from baseball to Spanish (Dom took an advanced placement test for De La Salle), to Shakespeare (he's reading "A Midsummer Night's Dream"), to flying Virgin America back from Washington, DC. We had such a great time and didn't get home until 10pm, but I know Mom loved every minute of it!

The next day, Thursday, May 8, I received news that I got the job! Oh, happy day! I'm the newest employee at Intervine Inc. as the Director of Sales for North America and Europe. I know my mom and my dad are happy for me, but Mom's already telling everyone she's losing her chauffeur, chef, and Girl Friday! I start work tomorrow – on Monday, May 12. So, once again there'll be some juggling and adjusting at home, but my hope is that in the end it helps Mom and Pop get back to living their lives the way they want to (and without a somewhat bossy daughter around 24/7). Ha!

So, coming full circle, today is Mother's Day and what a day it was. We went to church at 11 am and we were all together – Mom, Pop, me, Joe, Janine, Gab, and Dom. Just how Mom wanted it – surrounded by love on all sides. After church, we all went over to the Yountville Golf Course for lunch and had a great time on the patio. After lunch, we came home and I decided that my car needed to be washed in prep for my first day of work tomorrow. I tried to employ the help of Gab and Dom, but they were having none of it as long as their dad had possession of the hose.

See, it's been tradition over the years that Joe and I would always end up outside with my dad – surrendering with our hands up. My dad would have the hose and he'd threaten to spray us. Today, just like old times, it was Joe and I washing my car first and then his car with my dad watching from the sidelines. Of course, Joe plans for a little payback with the hose – but my dad was too smart for that. So, what does Joe do? He turned it on me! But not to worry, after we were done with Joe's car, Dom comes running up with a bucket of water and dumps it on Joe! Ha! Yes, payback...So much fun and full of antics this afternoon and, of course, Mom was enjoying herself from the sidelines and taking it all in. So, it was a nice and mellow day spent with the most important people in my life – my family.

Perhaps this Mother's Day is more meaningful and special to me because of all that Mom has endured these past six months. Yes, it has been a very long and tough six months. I'd say she's been to hell and back and for that, I'm eternally grateful to her for fighting. We have all wanted her to fight for her life even when she didn't want to have the surgery or the chemo. But she did it and she has truly handled all of this with the utmost grace and dignity.

I count my blessings for her (and my dad and my brother) every day. I realize that I won't always have my mom sitting next to me. In fact, I can't remember the last time I was actually home for Mother's Day. As I reflect on how many people don't have their mothers to share this day with, I must say that I definitely missed not having my grandmother here today as I know she would have added her two cents worth and gotten a kick out of all the antics!

In closing, yes, today is Mother's Day but it's

just one day. I try to honor my mother every day – knowing that I don't know how many more I will have with her. Of course, I pray we'll have many more years together and that Mom can soon start to enjoy again all that life has to offer and to do it on her terms. She certainly deserves that and so much more! That's my wish for Mom on this Mother's Day...and here's wishing all of you mothers out there a very special day surrounded by the love and kindness of your loved ones. HAPPY MOTHER'S DAY!

CHAPTER 12

THE CHOICES WE MAKE

Thursday, June 5

Opportunities and the Choices We Make

I'm sure you're wondering what's been going on, as it's been a few weeks without any update. I have no real good explanation other than I'm a full-time employee now and at the end of each day my head hurts from "information overload and a steep learning curve." Not to worry, as I do have many updates to share! I'll start by saying that it's been a bit of a rollercoaster – and leave it to Mom to keep us all on our toes!

I'll take you back to Sunday, May 18, when we had another lovely family gathering for Gabriella's high school graduation from Carondelet. I hate to admit how many years it's been since I graduated from CHS, so I won't. I'll continue to deny, deny,

deny. It was a truly special afternoon. What I remember most was Gab's beautiful smile. She's all grown up and now heading off to college – Cal Poly San Luis Obispo, here she comes! Go Mustangs! She'll be starting college this month for summer school and will get to meet and start practicing with her Mustang basketball teammates. It's a mandate for the student athletes and I think a great intro to the school and local vibe before all the other students arrive in September.

Then on Tuesday, May 20, it was a milestone day – Mom's last chemo treatment! 18 of 18 completed. I can't begin to tell you what a little dance I was doing in my own skin. I'm sure Mom didn't feel much different, but I could tell from the energy that day in the infusion room that we were all celebrating this little milestone. Making it extra special was my brother Joe escorting Mom to this last treatment, too. Yes, it was a family affair.

We brought in special treats from Bouchon Bakery (you know, Thomas Keller from French Laundry) for the entire staff – nurses, administrators, etc. Oh, and not to be left out are the AMAZING raisin and pecan scones from the pastry chef at R+D. Hint: they are only sold at Kelly's (a little gas station/coffee and retail shop) in Yountville and sell out by noon each day. That's an inside local scoop.

I'd say we definitely got the morning off to a great

start. And once at the treatment center, the nurses surprised Mom with a certificate and three delicious cupcakes from a delectable Napa bakery.

Theresa, the head nurse, held true to her promise. Mom and I remember the first day we met her – she promised us that she'd get Mom through this. I can tell you that I probably gave her the questionable evil eye, as I was highly doubtful about anything back then. But she was right…she got Mom through it all.

Then, Mom and I decided to do a little celebration of our own and we ventured over to Bistro Jeanty in Yountville for lunch…Mom's favorite dish: the Petrale Sole with mashed potatoes. And I had the mussels in a savory wine sauce, and it was fabulous as always. Next best thing to being in Paris!

A week would soon pass, as I had arranged a little "vacation" to check out and give myself some down time before the job really kicked in. In fact, I think this was the first vacation I'd ever taken by myself. I went to Belize, and it was just what I needed…a little relaxation in my hammock overlooking the beautiful Caribbean Sea and taking in that lovely tropical breeze. I got back on May 27 and then the whirlwind began.

Aunt Beth and Mom had tickets to see Johnny Mathis in concert, so we made it a mother/daughter evening. Aunt Beth, my cousin Terri, Mom, and I met in Sonoma for dinner and then ventured over to Marin Civic Center to see the swooner in concert. What a night…I gotta give it to the guy – he still has it going on. I remember Mom listening to his records (yes, records in those days) and especially his Christmas album. One thing I realized about Johnny Mathis was that he sang a lot of ballads and romantic songs.

Needless to say, he still made Mom's heart flutter still – and in more ways than you can imagine! Which leads me to this next story.

So, the next day, I knew that Mom had to be exhausted. We didn't get home until after midnight and I knew she'd not been feeling very well. I had to go to work that day, but around 4:15pm I got a call from Mom (I've learned to always keep my cell phone with me in case of an emergency). She was having trouble and thought she was in a-fib (which she was). I'll give her this – she is definitely in tune with how she feels and knew that this was somewhat of concern. So, I rushed home and my dad and I were there with her to assess the situation. Once I took her blood pressure, we knew there was a problem.

Long story short, we had to call the paramedics and get some help. They took Mom to the hospital, and she remained there for two days for tests, X-ray, blood work, etc. Once again, her amazing doctors came through. She'd spoken with Dr. Jewell (her GP) and Dr. Dugan (her oncologist) somehow found out she was there, and he popped in to check on Mom. And of course, Mom's little angel at Queen of the Valley, Terri Gardella, came by to have lunch with mom and pay her a visit. So, as usual, she was in great hands. Mom needed a blood transfusion for some extra red blood cells along with a Neupogen shot to boost her white blood cells as well. But hey, I'm just going to chalk all this up to Johnny still making Mom's heart go aflutter!

The major downside to all this was that Mom missed Dom's graduation from the eighth grade at St. Mary's School. While she was resting in the hospital, the rest of my family and I joined Dom for his very special day. I gotta tell ya, I never had an eighth-grade graduation like that. It was so nice, and what a wonderful ceremony. We saw Dom receive his diploma and even win The Spirit Award – given to a student who displays not only academic excellence, but always lends a helping hand and is generous towards his fellow classmates. One of the most interesting aspects of his graduation ceremony was the fact that they had a guest speaker. And this year it was Coach Bob Ladoucer (teacher and football coach at De La Salle High School). I'll get to that speech in a little bit…after the graduation ceremony we took photos and I texted them all to Mom, so she could feel like she was there too.

Then, on Saturday, May 31, Mom was released

from the hospital (I think she probably threatened a doc or two) because she was determined to get to the party. You know Mom, she's always one for a party! It was a joint graduation party for Gab and Dom at Joe and Janine's house. And what a day it was! I personally loved the margarita machine (yes, they even had some Gran Marnier floating in there!) and fabulous food. Joe has the perfect house for an outdoor gathering, and it was a revolving door all afternoon, into the evening, and apparently until 1:30 am for a late-night extravaganza of steaks and who knows what else! Mom was tuckered out, so we headed out and got back home around 9pm.

Up until today, she's been resting and taking it easy – and I think Mom's feeling a little better each day. In fact, this afternoon it was a Fab 5 reunion to celebrate Donna's birthday and I know Mom was really looking forward to seeing all her girlfriends. And next up on Mom's radar is another party (of course!). Mom is co-hosting a baby shower with Mayra for Connie's new grandson-to-be. It's going to be a fabulous afternoon English tea. It is in full force planning mode, and I think it's just what Mom needs to keep her spirits up and it's also something wonderful to look forward to.

In closing, I'll now digress back to Coach Lad, and his speech at Dom's graduation. For those of you not familiar with Coach Lad, I believe he's the most winning coach of all time. (In fact, there's a book that was published about him and his legacy, as well as a movie on the big screen, "When the Game Stands Tall." But the takeaway here was in Coach Lad's message. It was truly engaging and poignant – his portrayal and description of what these eighth graders will encounter on this next life-changing chapter. What resonated with me the most was the correlation he made between the opportunities we have in life and the decisions and choices we make along the way. And I will bring this back full circle to Mom's journey.

Mom, too, has had many opportunities and choices to make these past eight months – to have surgery or not, to do traditional chemo or not, to have a positive mental outlook or not, to venture out and make time to be at basketball and baseball games or not, to eat healthy or not. And I could go on and on. But these are all choices that she has had to make. And I do believe that the opportunities she has created for herself are a direct reflection of all the positive choices that she has made.

The end result is a life well-lived with so many incredible memories shared with family and friends – even through the toughest of times. And I envision a bright future ahead for Mom with so much more living to do…and I hope she sees it that way, too. May we always remember that we are a direct reflection of the choices we make. So, here's to living life in a positive and meaningful way no matter what challenges life throws at you!

Friday, July 25
Embarking on a New Journey

It's Friday, and I've been remiss about not keeping you all up to date on Mom's latest and greatest adventures. I'm happy to report all good news – her latest check up with her oncologist Dr. Dugan this month was a glowing report (her CA-125 marker is where it should be!). And her visit to Dr. Lerner, her surgeon, was also incredibly positive. In fact, he was quite surprised to see that Mom drove herself down to Walnut Creek for the appointment. Sort of makes me chuckle to myself...

I remember very vividly that day last October – let's call it "The Inquisition" – with this renowned surgeon. The Grupalo clan showed up to meet this young surgeon and hear from him firsthand about what this journey would entail. I'm sure we all looked like deer caught in the headlights just trying to make sense of it all and comprehend what he was saying. While we all knew that it was Mom "flying solo" on this mission, we made it very clear from the start that we would all be there for her – each of us in our own special way. And yes, I'm delighted to report that my dad, Joe, and I have stuck by her side since that first day we learned of her cancer diagnosis nine months ago.

It has been a very long and winding road, but here she is getting stronger and stronger each day.

Here's the beauty in this – everyone did their part – and now...well, Dolly is back!

She's kickin' up her heels (well, sort of) and is in full force and living life on her terms and loving every minute of it again! I can't begin to tell you all the lunches, dinners, events, outings, and games that she's been going to. It's a bit overwhelming, even for me! She doesn't stop (and who can blame her?) and I think she's pickin' up the pace. Her dance card is full!

And this week marks a very special time – while I sit here writing this, she is enjoying her first road trip! She has flown the coop! The wheels are in motion and she's down at Cal Poly San Luis Obispo with my dad, Joe, Janine, Gabriella, and Dom. Gab just finished summer school and basketball training (she'll be a freshman this fall), so they were all down there this week to move her out of the dorm and spend some quality time exploring the area and Avila Beach.

So, I guess you could ask the question, "Was it all worth it?"

Without hesitation, my answer is YES. (I'm hoping she would agree with me). To see the joy, happiness, and love emanating from Mom is priceless. The pictures of her now really reflect the Dolly we all know and remember. Her smile is much wider, the skip in her step a little bigger, there's a brighter twinkle in her eye, a louder and more joyous laugh, and the hugs are a bit more forceful (she is definitely gaining her strength back)!

Tomorrow, Mom and I will be participating in the Relay for Life – yes, it'll be a glorious day to celebrate how far she has come (and kicked cancer to the curb!) on this not-so-fun journey.

Ultimately, I think this is why we fight – to be with the ones we love, to have more quality time together, and to create more wonderful, lasting memories each and every day for as long as we can.

So, on that note, I will announce that I'll be taking some time off from this journal.

In closing, I want to give special thanks to my dad and my brother for being there through it all (the good, the bad, and all the in between). Your unwavering commitment to our family has also helped me immensely and is a truly cherished blessing. To all you readers out there – friends and family – your incredible gifts of prayer, friendship, and love through this journey are so incredibly appreciated. Your support is what has sustained all of us through this trying time. A huge shout out goes to all the amazing doctors and nurses who have helped Mom through surgery, chemo, and beyond. The care was first-rate and the positive outlook you instilled made a lasting impact with Mom. Jeni, you will always have a special place in her heart!

And finally, my biggest heartfelt thank you goes out to Mom. Thank you for fighting – especially when you didn't want to. Thank you for trying and believing. Thank you for eating my healthy food (I know you still want your sugar). Thank you for trying to meditate, take a few extra walks here and there, and do all the little things I hoped would help. I'm such a believer in treating our health with a comprehensive mind, body, and spirit approach. I left nothing to chance. You did all I asked and so much more. I cherish each and every day with you and look forward to all the new memories that you'll be creating with me and all those who are near and dear to you. May you embrace and cherish each day for what it is – a very special gift! ILYMTT

Tuesday, September 23
A Very Special Day!

Three days ago, Mom, Pop, and I ventured out to Pittsburg to watch Dom's baseball game – De La Salle Fall baseball is under way! It's so fun to watch him in action – he's so confident – and to see him in that Spartan green! After the game, we all went to lunch at Stanford's in Walnut Creek. It was Dom's pick and so perfect, as that is where Dom and Mom would always go to lunch together when she babysat him in his younger years….to wrap it up, what a whirlwind weekend! And it didn't end there.

Last night, Mom and Pop went over to Santa Rosa for dinner and a fabulous evening with Aunt Beth and Uncle Keith. The party continues.

I am writing and posting this today because it is indeed a very special day...today is Mom's birthday! I'm guessing it's going to be one of the most meaningful and memorable birthdays ever. It's a true blessing and one that I know comes with much heartfelt appreciation to everyone who has stood by her side this past year to offer up support in so many ways – prayers, hugs, phone calls, cards, visits, food delivery, and so much love to go around!

When I was in Italy earlier this month with Gabriella, I said at least one prayer for Mom in every church I went to. I'm sure you can imagine how many that was! And at The Vatican and St. Peter's Basilica, there were extra prayers said. One of my wishes has certainly come true – Mom is here today and living her life to the fullest. She's got her partners in crime (I am just one of many) and there is absolutely no slowing her down! So much more of life to embrace and how sweet it is today – HAPPY BIRTHDAY, MOM! ILYMTT

CHAPTER 13

WEDDING CRASHERS

A follow up visit with Dr. Lerner is nothing out of the ordinary until Mom comes home to report that Dr. Lerner is getting married in September – in the Napa Valley.

"That's great, Mom. I'm sure he'll have a lovely wedding in the fall."

"Well, I asked him when the date is, what time the ceremony is, and where he's going to have the reception. He says no patients will be invited, but I told him that I wanted to come. And he said that was fine."

"Mom, of course he said it would be fine. What else could he say to you? He was trying to be considerate and polite."

Of course, he should have known better than to leak his wedding details to Mom. Had I not warned him before? Too late – before I knew it, Mom had recruited me to be her driver and accomplice. She was now planning to crash the surgeon's wedding!

Worried that we may cause a scene and get kicked out of this very intimate wedding, I threw my hands up.

"Oh, well," I said. "It's your surgeon and you can bail us out of whatever you get us into."

Once again, I did warn him about her.

A sweltering September Saturday afternoon in the valley has us both uncomfortable. Wearing our best dress and with my face painted on (did I mention that I'm not big on makeup?), I'm already sweating. But it's worse for Mom, because she's also got her wig to contend with. And apparently, they don't breathe well. Although I told her to wear the wig with the shortest amount of hair, she's literally sweating from head to toe. To add to our misery, the traffic today is unrelenting. Tourists are everywhere leisurely cruising up and down the valley in search of wineries and tasting rooms. And it is harvest time! You can always tell the tourists, because they drive at a snail's pace trying to take photos and check out the views along the way while we locals are zipping around trying get to our destinations.

Adding another layer of complexity is the fundraiser bike ride taking place, which is causing major delays due to road closures and diversions. Behind the wheel, Mom was on a mission to get us there on time. I am fully cursing Mom under my breath because she is rarely on time but it's a special day, so I suggest we opt for the scenic Silverado Trail as we inch our way north to Calistoga. Forty-five minutes later, we pulled into Solage Resort.

With just a few minutes to spare, we find our way and

are surrounded with simple elegance. It's serene with charming cottages strewn throughout the property. We make our way to the outdoor venue and are greeted by a lush garden where plants, trees, and greenery are plentiful. The gilded chairs are lined up in rows, each side separated by the center aisle. People are handing out parasols to help beat the heat. I can see Mom scanning the crowd to see if there's anyone here she knows. While I've instructed Mom to hang back and just try to blend in among the guests, she proudly states that we are here on behalf of the groom and would like to be seated.

Parasols and little handheld misters helped to battle the heat (which was not really that hot in my Las Vegas opinion) and, yes, they had enough chairs for us to sit down. After the ceremony, we continued to crash the pre-reception party. We saw Dr. Edraki there (the other brilliant surgeon who assisted in Mom's surgery) and also Mojdeh Palmer, the office manager, who continues to always make time for Mom and has been so incredibly helpful. Everyone, of course, commented on how fabulous Mom looked and I personally think she should be the new "poster woman" for their practice!

Well, of course, after hanging out long enough, I knew exactly what Mom was up to. There was no way she was leaving without saying "Congratulations" to Dr. Lerner. So, of course, Mom inches her way over (quite gracefully, I might add) to Dr. Lerner and he just lit up at seeing her. He gave her a huge hug and his first comment was how beautiful Mom looked. Yes, she was radiant! We gave our quick "congrats" to the bride and groom, and then headed out for a great little sushi dinner. Perfect ending to a great wedding crasher day!

Thursday, November 13
One Year Post Surgery

Today is a day that our family is certainly celebrating and perhaps each of us in his or her own way. It's not a birthday, an anniversary, or a job promotion.

Can you believe it was exactly one year ago today that Mom had her life-changing (and saving) surgery? My how time flies! It's sure been a bumpy ride, but today that road is smooth and there is joy in all our hearts knowing we have all come so far.

Mom is doing GREAT (to say the least) and she continues to live each day with pure joy, happiness, gratitude, and love in her heart. You can't help but see it, feel it, and notice it – that sparkle in her eyes is back and shining even brighter. She appreciates each day for what it is – a gift – and she definitely practices what she preaches.

Her days are quite filled with all sorts of fun activities – attending the World Series to see the San Francisco Giants (Game 5); riding her bike through the vineyards with Elizabeth Swanson (her first bike ride in over a year!); lunches and dinners with my dad, Uncle Keith, Aunt Beth, her Fab 5 friends, and her Tap Sisters; and the list goes on and on. I've also given Mom three tickets to see a film tomorrow at the Napa Valley Film Festival called "What the F@# Is Cancer and Why Does Everybody Have It"? she's going to attend with two of her friends, Carol Fink and Jaime Hunt – all three of them are cancer survivors! My heart goes out to all three ladies and I hope that they have a wonderful time together celebrating the life that each of them has fought (and continue to fight) so hard for. There's no stopping Mom now...jump on that wagon and join her for a fabulous ride! Just say "yes" and be an accomplice to whatever the adventure...you most certainly won't be disappointed!

I can honestly say that I love being back home and spending time with my parents and Joe and his family. The pain and dark days are truly bright again. Instead of dwelling on the past and what ifs, I'm focusing on today. And I know Mom is, too. She's got a busy day planned for herself...how appropriate that she has a follow up appointment today with her surgeon Dr. Lerner.

This is how special a doctor he is to her – Mom said to me this morning, "What am I going to do when he no longer needs to see me?" I know she really enjoys her time with him and that she considers him a friend and an integral part of her "Special Ops" team. I told her that she should continue to make her "appointments" and that there's no way he would refuse to see her. In fact, I'm sure it's good for his soul, too. Knowing Mom, she'll remind him of how special today is and give her thanks for the amazing doctor he is and for the special relationship that they share.

And if this doesn't give you chills, I don't know what will. Would you believe that literally as I'm writing this blog, I receive a most beautiful floral arrangement? And who from...Mom, of course! That is just the kind of woman she is...thanking me for helping her. When here I am saying "thank you" to her for believing in herself as well as her family to help see her through the depths of despair of death knocking on her door. And for believing that one day the sun would shine again for her and there would be life worth living.

Here's to your one-year anniversary, Mom – and to living this life on your terms. May it bring you all the joy, love, and happiness you wish for. I know those stars will definitely be shining bright tonight!

Wednesday, January 28, 2015
Checking It Off the Bucket List
Greetings and Happy New Year to all! I couldn't resist checking in and sharing this news with everyone this evening.

Today, while I was sitting in my office busy at work, I received a text message from Mom with some news.

It is the sort of news that stops you in your tracks – in a good way. How often does that happen? I literally found myself sitting back in my chair soaking in each and every word that she had written. I was overwhelmed with gratitude, joy, and happiness hearing about the "bucket list day," as I'm calling it. It's hard to explain what I was feeling, but there was a warmth and contentment knowing that this was one of those moments that made this tough journey so worthwhile.

In its essence, this email that I'm about to share with you is about believing in yourself, overcoming the odds, and persevering to finish on top...doing the things you love to do! Now, the game may have changed a bit – but it's clear that Mom has definitely adapted. As I keep trying to tell her, you have to embrace change. It's certainly not easy, but can be so incredibly rewarding – as today certainly was. Without further ado, here's the email, exactly as I received it today (punctuation and all!):

Hi Nan, today is a "historical" day for me!! 14 months after major surgery and 12 months after starting chemotherapy and 8 months after having completed chemo, I was out on the tennis courts!! It was an absolutely beautiful cool but sunny winter day! (And my wig didn't fall off - and my thigh high compression hose didn't fall down - and I didn't fall down - so all of that was great!) My tennis skills were not great - in fact were very rusty but it was soooo great just to be out there!! Thank YOU for helping me get to this "bucket list" activity! ILYMTT!! Mom

Now if that doesn't inspire you, what will? What I do know is that Mom has been wanting to get back out on the tennis court, but was trepidatious about her possible physical limitations as well as any possible other malfunctions (wig-related or otherwise). I told her that if Andre Agassi could play in the U.S. Open with a hairpiece and not be rattled, she could too! She had a lesson today with her former coach, Rick, and her teammate, Nancy Gardner. Now, Mom may have been slower than before and, apparently, she hit a few air balls – but hey, that's ok. It can only get better and at least she was out there! How great is that?

The beauty in this message for me is seeing her determination, will, and strength to continue doing the things that bring her the most joy. And there is such joy and happiness in this text. It made my heart sing! And I suspect that there's even more joy than I can imagine in this momentous occasion, given the journey she's had to endure to finally arrive here.

So, my message to all – remember this day and what it represents. May you embrace and live each day to the fullest – stay the course and don't let the obstacles get in your way or hold you back. You have the power to make it happen! And may you also be able to check off whatever it is on your bucket list. Oh, and Mom just told me tonight that she is already plotting her next goal (it must be the next item on her bucket list)...DANCING!

CHAPTER 14

IRELAND

Since my mother's diagnosis almost two years ago, I have repeatedly inquired, "Mom, what else would you like to do in your life once you get through surgery and your chemo treatments? Anything special you want to do? Here is what I propose: I want to honor you and take you on a very special trip – anywhere in the world you want to go. You get to pick the place. It will be a way for us to celebrate all that you have been through and for being here today."

Her response has always been one and the same, "I am doing exactly what I have wanted to do. Most important is to share my time with family, friends, and loved ones. I don't need anything special, and I don't need to travel to far and distant places anymore. I'm most content to visit the places that have become the most comfortable and meaningful to me."

And I know those places that she is referring to – the

shores of Maui and the mountains of Montana. And everywhere in between, which usually happens to be wherever Gab is playing in the latest Cal Poly women's basketball game or where Dom is hitting and fielding with the De La Salle varsity baseball team.

I have learned from my mother that the simple joys in life are often the most endearing and heartfelt. And so, I, too, now have my list of favorite places to visit where I find peace and joy within. And that apple sure didn't fall far from the tree – as my true inherent happiness is also found wherever my friends and family are, especially my niece and nephew.

But then one day, months later and completely out of the blue, Mom says to me, "I think I know where I would like to go."

And with confusion, I ask her, "Go where? For what trip?"

She replies, "You know, the trip that you promised we could take. I want to go to Ireland!"

"Ireland? Why do you want to go to Ireland? We aren't even Irish?"

And with passports in hand, our adventures will continue…across the pond and over to Ireland in 2015. Just a mother and daughter exploring and celebrating life together, one precious moment at a time.

EPILOGUE

Almost 10 years have passed since that life-altering diagnosis. My, how time flies. In early March 2020, I hit the trifecta – moved to Atlanta, started a new job, and Covid struck. All alone in a new city where I didn't know anyone, my coping mechanism was soon found in the joy and comfort through the eyes and energy of Lexi, my new goldendoodle puppy. For Mom, however, I sensed her coping mechanism was in her friends and family.

As I am writing this, it is now 2023. Mom remains in good health, and she continues to embrace the sunrise and sunset of each day and every moment in between. We all know our days are numbered – but for her, I can tell it resonates just a little deeper. There is a renewed appreciation for time, and she does not take one day for granted. Today, we both live and experience life a little more intently, intentionally, and with purpose.

Yes, life has continued to move forward – but it has been shrouded in more loss and illness of those nearest and dearest. Mom has not only lost a sister and a brother unexpectedly, but she has also mourned the loss of dear friends which span her lifetime since childhood. Equally difficult and heartbreaking is enduring the process as one by one, her friends battle with dementia, Alzheimer's, and ALS. If there is one thing the aging process has taught me, it is not for the faint of heart. Illness and disease are just one degree of separation away. So, how will we choose to spend our time? And what will we decide to focus our energy on?

For Mom, life has always been deeply rooted in family and friends. Her guiding light has always been and continues to be led by a devotion to her faith, family, and friends. In retrospect, I believe this guiding light has served her well and been the foremost contributor to her recovery and being alive today. Against all odds, she has won the battle and lives each day in celebration.

Her days are planned and filled with activities – Wednesday afternoons are for Mahjong; Thursday evenings are for card playing and champagne drinking with her "tap sisters"; and every morning is a Wordle competition among Mom, Joe, and me to see who reigns with a crown for the day. Her dance card is full – always. She continues to invest her precious time in family. And in her friends – even when those days of conversation and visual recognition have passed. She still shows up and is present, forever grateful for the bonds of friendship that have endured the test of time, illness, and suffering.

I recently received a phone call from Mom.

"I've been thinking; did you know it's our 10-year cancer-free anniversary this year? (Yes, of course, I knew.) And this time I would like to take you on a trip – wherever you want to go."

Speechless and totally surprised, the tears came to the surface. And although I had no words at that precise moment, I could feel my heart swell with gratitude and love. As you can probably imagine, it didn't take me long to energetically pitch my plan.

"Yes, let's celebrate with a new adventure. Are you comfortable traveling over the pond? What do you think about taking a Christmas on the Rhine River cruise?"

I feel as though we have come full circle, managing the commodity of time. Looking forward, a new adventure awaits. Mom has just renewed her passport. Europe is calling.

FURTHER READING

Some readers of this book may also find themselves struggling and unsure of how to manage an unexpected illness as a patient or as a caregiver. If that is you, here are a few resources that helped me. Perhaps, they will help you too. May they empower you with knowledge, get you thinking in a different way, ask questions you never thought of, provide comfort of the unknown, and inspire you to live a more compassionate and meaningful life.

- CaringBridge.org
- National Ovarian Cancer Coalition (NOCC) – ovarian.org
- Ovarian Cancer Research Alliance (OCRA) – ocrahope.org
- Cancer.org
- Wellbeingjournal.com (Vol. 23, No. 2): "Sugar, Cancer and Disease Prevention" article by Mark Sircus, OMD
- Anti-Cancer – A New Way of Life by Dr. David Servan-Schreiber
- Into the Magic Shop by Dr. James R. Doty
- The Caregiver's Prayer by Ron Cooper

ACKNOWLEDGMENTS

To Mom, Pop, and Joe, my deepest heartfelt gratitude goes to you for making this book possible, as we lived this story together. Mom and Pop, you opened the door for me to come home and let me take the reins during an incredibly challenging time. Your unconditional love, support, and quiet strength helped me to stay the course and just do what needed to be done. And Joe, you are still the one I choose to have in the foxhole with me.

To Gab and Dom, thank you for lighting up my life and helping me to smile, especially when I wasn't feeling it. You bring tremendous joy, love, and happiness to my life and inspire me to be the best version of myself. I love you dearly!

Aunt Beth and Keith, thank you! I'll always remember that you were by my side from the very beginning—through the entire surgery, the visit to ICU, and every activity, sporting event, and family gathering thereafter.

And to my cousin Jerri, your positive attitude, uplifting energy, and outpouring of love is contagious. You will always have a special place in my heart!

To Dr. Dimitry Lerner, Dr. Babak Edraki, Dr. Paul Dugan, Dr. David Freeto, Dr. Benjamin Jewell, Jeni-Lee Burke, Teresa Dugan, and all the doctors, nurses, and caregivers who have given of themselves to help Mom fight her battle with cancer, I give special thanks! Through your life's mission, you have provided strength, comfort, and care when it was most needed. And you did so in the most gracious and humane manner possible. You have saved a life and for that, I am eternally grateful.

I am incredibly grateful to my editor, Stephanie Mojica. You provided light at the end of the tunnel when I didn't see it and brought this book to life. Your encouragement truly kindled a spark that this story had merit and was one worth sharing. Your brilliance shines through!

To Asya Blue, my book illustrator and format editor, thank you for bringing this cover to life and capturing the true essence of my vision in color and design. I am so impressed and forever grateful for your guidance along the way and to bring it all together. Your work is genius!

And to Bill Rogoway and Carol Fink, thank you for honoring me and taking the time to read through this manuscript before anyone else laid eyes on it.

To the "Tap and Step Sisters" (aka Dolly's Dancers), your paths crossed years ago over a mutual love for tap dancing. And your friendship has endured long beyond your tap-dancing days. I'm incredibly grateful to each of you, as you were there for Mom through every "shuffle ball change" and "time step" of the way.

And thank you to Mom's friends from every walk of life. Your friendships have truly stood the test of time: Alleman High School (Rock Island, IL), Mercy School of Nursing at St. Ambrose University (Davenport, IA), St. Perpetua Parishioners (Lafayette, CA), The Fab 5 and Razzamatazz Players (Walnut Creek, CA), and the St. Joan of Arc Parishioners (Yountville, CA).

To my wonderful lifeline of friends, colleagues and acquaintances I've met along this journey, THANK YOU! You helped to prop me up on my darkest days and brought a little humor, laughter, and peace into my heart. You provided kindness and gentle guidance when needed and a shoulder to lean on when I couldn't manage on my own. Your unconditional love and enduring friendship across state lines and country borders is a truly cherished and precious gift. I hope that someday I can do the same for you and be that shoulder to lean on, provide the hug you need, and be a loving friend to help you manage through whatever life throws your way. Heartfelt appreciation and gratitude go out to Carla Alston, Sylvie Rathier, Chris Cappas, Kristine Mastrodonato, Chris Flatt, Christine Brzysko, Bridget Moloney, Sharna Brockett, Andrew Junius, Amy Lilley, Anne Garsztka, Chris Maulsby, Karen Bennett, Patsy McGaughy, Jack Marx, Parasto Niakian, Michael Borck, Ed Matovcik, Michelle Few, Shany Cruz, Kim Stone, April Harmon, Summer Seret, Susan Cady, and Albert Repola.

To Shawna Terry and Gary Patrick Gemma, thank you both for your incredible support and guidance on how best to lose one's hair gracefully. With a glass of Champagne, of course!

To Julie Nelson, Regan Lawson, Beth Moore, and Lauren Bucci you are the dearest friends a California transplant to Georgia could ever hope for. Thank you for your most precious gift of friendship and for your continued encouragement to get this book across the finish line. Love you guys!

In honor and special memory of Rose Solis who left this world much too soon. Since her passing in 2022, Pancha's has remained closed. However, I like to think that Rose's spirit lives on, encouraging us to dance on any bar!

In closing, I am eternally grateful to the friends and family whose idea it was to turn this blog into a book. Over the course of three years from 2013-2016, I took that inspiration to heart and wrote this book. But then it sat dormant, collecting dust on a thumb drive for years. Finally, in 2023, a little internal spark nudged me to cross the finish line and bring this story to publication. It is in honor of Mom's milestone achievement and miracle—being free of ovarian cancer for 10 years. Cheers!

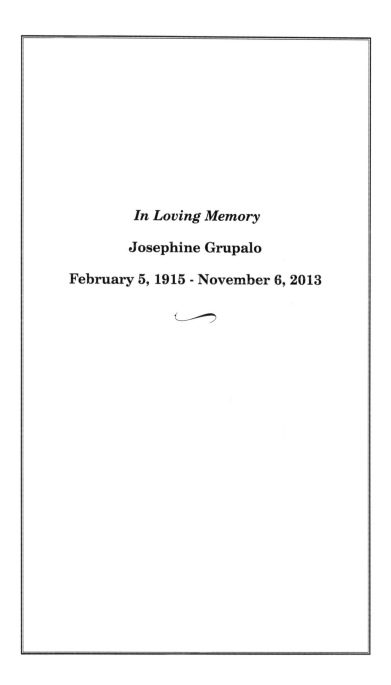

In Loving Memory

Josephine Grupalo

February 5, 1915 - November 6, 2013

PHOTOS

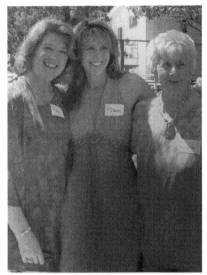

With Mom and Nonni (2005)

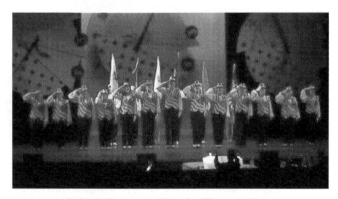

Dolly's Dancers, Lincoln Theater, Napa
(mom is 5th from the right) (March 2010)

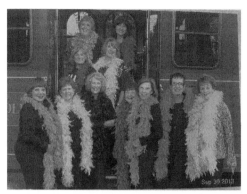

Dolly's Dancers enjoy a night out at Pancha's (September, 2013)
(top to bottom, left to right): Connie Courtright, Darlene de
Beauclair, Andrea Biocca, Dolly Grupalo, Mayra McKinney,
Joanne Hatch, Kathy Phillips, JoAnn Myers, Marlene Frappia,
Gretchen Oertel, Darlene Bevin)

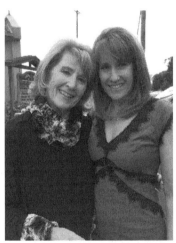

At Nonni's funeral, also the
day before surgery
(November 12, 2013)

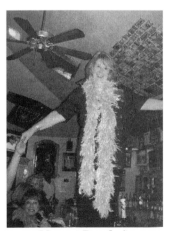

Mom at Pancha's,
dancing on the bar
(September 30, 2013)

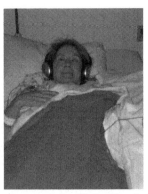

Mom is a patient at John Muir Hospital trying out
noise canceling headphones (November 2013)

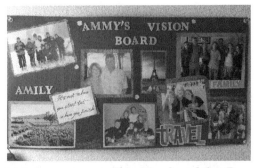

The vision board that Dom
and Gab created for Mom; it
hung in her hospital room and
later at home (with time it has
faded and missing a letter)
(November 2013)

With Gab after one of her
high school basketball games
(March 2014)

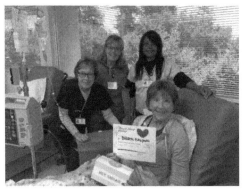

Mom celebrating her last chemo treatment
(May 20, 2014)

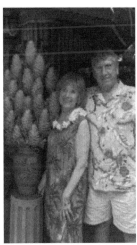

My parents, at Mama's
Fish House in Maui
(September 2014)

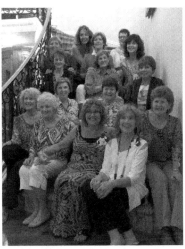

Dolly's Dancers gather together to
celebrate Mom's first post-cancer
birthday (September 2014)

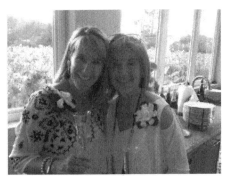

*Mom and I celebrating together
(September 2014)*

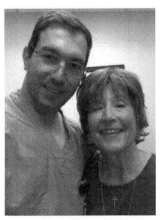

*Dr. Lerner and Mom on her one-year
post-surgery visit (November 2014)*

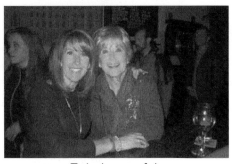

*Enjoying a pub in
Dublin, Ireland (April 2015)*

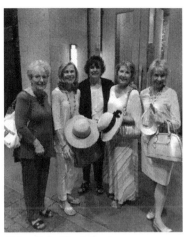

"The Fab 5" – Mom's group of friends for almost 50 years (August 2015) (l to r: Carol Scott, Donna Lindholm, Marianne Lamberts, Dolly Grupalo, Sheilah Morrison)

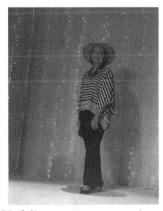

Modeling as a cancer survivor in "Reach for the Stars", a cancer fundraiser and benefit (April 2017)

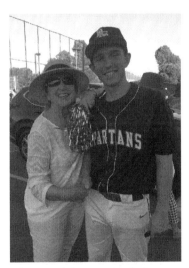

Mom is celebrating with Dom after one of his high school baseball games (May 2018)

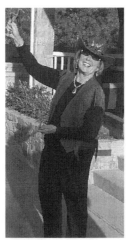

Mom celebrates 5-years
cancer free (October 2018)

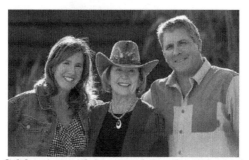

Celebrating with Mom and Joe (October 2018)

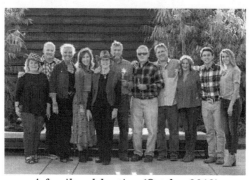

A family celebration (October 2018)

About Lizann Grupalo

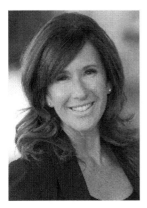

Lizann Grupalo grew up in Northern California. She earned a BA in Italian from Santa Clara University and her MBA in International Business from Middlebury Institute of International Studies at Monterey, Fisher Graduate School of Business.

A career in international business development and sales along with her entrepreneurial and adventurous spirit has encouraged her to live greatly and explore the world. The Commodity of Time is her first book. She lives in Alpharetta, Georgia with her mini goldendoodle Lexi.

About Dolly Grupalo

Dolly Grupalo was born in Rock Island, Illinois. She earned her bachelor's degree in nursing (BSN) from St. Ambrose University in Davenport, Iowa.

Upon graduation and in search of her own adventure, she made her way out West and settled in Northern California. After a successful and meaningful nursing career, Dolly focused on her love of tennis and tap dancing. She formed Dolly's Dancers where she taught tap and performed locally for 23 years. Today, she remains a vibrant part of her local community, is a loving wife to Don, a mother, an aunt, a grandmother, and a friend to many.

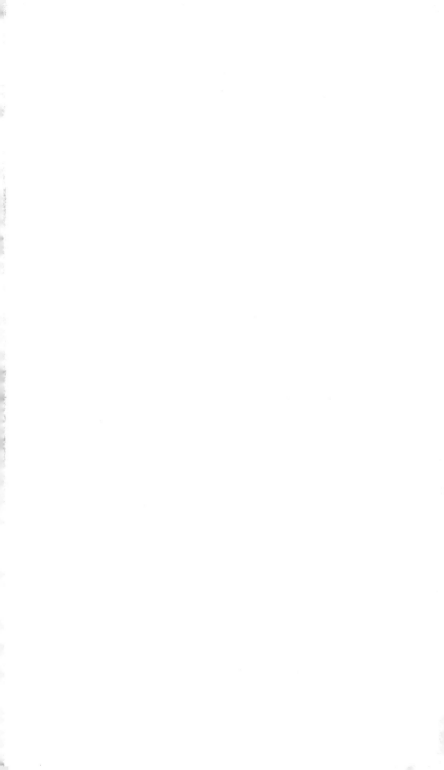

Made in the USA
Columbia, SC
19 February 2024

31798072R00140